Practice Papers
for the
DCH Examination

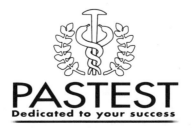

Practice Papers for the DCH Examination

Dr Jacqueline A Lynch
MBBS MRCS Ed (A&E) DCH DRCOG
Clinical Fellow, Intensive Care,
Queen Alexandra Hospital,
Portsmouth.

Edited by

Dr I Pollock
Consultant Paediatrician
Chase Farm Hospital,
Enfield, Middlesex.

Clinical section by

Dr R M Beattie
Consultant Paediatrician
Southampton General Hospital,
Tremona Road,
Southampton, Hampshire.

© 2000 PASTEST
Egerton Court
Parkgate Estate
Knutsford
Cheshire WA16 8DX

Telephone: 01565 752000

First published 2000
Reprinted 2002

ISBN 1 901198 52 9

A catalogue record for this book is available from the British Library.

PasTest Revision Books and Intensive Courses
PasTest has been established in the field of postgraduate medical education since 1972, providing revision books and intensive study courses for doctors preparing for their professional examinations.
Books and courses are available for the following specialties:
MRCP Part 1 and Part 2, MRCPCH Part 1 and Part 2, MRCOG, DRCOG, MRCGP, MRCPsych, DCH, FRCA, MRCS, PLAB.
For further details contact:
**PasTest, Freepost, Knutsford, Cheshire WA16 7BR
Tel: 01565 752000   Fax: 01565 650264
E-mail: enquiries@pastest.co.uk
Web site: www.pastest.co.uk**

Typeset by Breeze Ltd, Manchester.
Printed by Bell & Bain Ltd., Glasgow

CONTENTS

ACKNOWLEDGEMENTS

I would like to thank all my family and friends for their help with this publication, especially Dr. Kirsty Adams, Dr. Kelly Forbes, Ms Lucy Vinter and Mrs Marion Vinter.

I would like to dedicate this book to Niall, Barry and Jamie and particularly my mother and father whose unwavering love, support and occasional threats have always helped me to succeed when failure would have been a lot easier!

Jacqueline A Lynch

NOTES ON PASSING THE DCH EXAM

The majority of candidates in the UK sit the Diploma of Child Health examination run by the Royal College of Paediatrics and Child Health. It is designed to give recognition of competence in the care of children to General Practitioner vocational trainees, Staff Grades and SHOs in paediatrics and trainees in specialties allied to paediatrics. The aim is to test primary care paediatrics, especially from the following aspects: Epidemiology, Prenatal Care, Nutrition & Feeding, Growth & Development, Immunisation & Screening, Health Surveillance & Promotion, Accident Prevention, Child Abuse and Legislation, as well as the diagnosis and management of the principal childhood conditions.

THE EXAMINATION

Candidates are advised to have completed a minimum of six months experience of Paediatrics and Child Health before sitting the examination as it is unlikely that a candidate would be successful without this experience.

Candidates who have passed either the MRCP (UK) Part 1 examination or Part 1 of the MRCPCH within the previous seven years are exempt from Written Paper 1 of the DCH Examination.

The examination consists of two sections:
*   **Written section** containing two papers
    Paper 1 –   60 MCQs (two hours)
    Paper 2 –   (three hours) 10 Short Note Cases (which account for 50% of the total marks)
                2 Case Commentaries (each case accounts for 25% of the total marks).

Candidates must pass Paper 1 in order to attend the Clinical Session. Answers to Written Paper 2 are not marked where candidates have gained insufficient marks in Paper 1.

Paper 1 and 2 are held on the same day, if candidates are successful they will be invited to attend the Clinical Examination held approximately 4–5 weeks later.

- **Clinical section** consists of
  One Long Case – 40 minutes with the patient and 20 minutes discussion.
  Short Cases – 30 minutes total of which 10 minutes will be devoted to developmental testing, including the testing of vision/hearing.

NB. The Written Paper 2 and Long and Short Cases have individual pass marks. A failure in either the Long or Short Case cannot be compensated by a good performance in other sections and will result in an overall fail in the examination. A Bare Fail in Written Paper 2 can be compensated by a good performance in either the Long or Short Case.

THE WRITTEN PAPERS

Multiple Choice Questions
There are 60 questions each having 5 stems which are either 'True' or 'False'. One mark (+) will be awarded for each correct answer and a zero mark will be awarded for each 'Don't Know' (D) response. From September 2000 negative marking has been abolished.

Remember to read each stem carefully and look out for terms such as 'always/never' (GENERALLY False) and 'may/can' (GENERALLY True).

Short Note Questions
It is recommended that half your time should be spent on the Short Note Questions. There are 10 questions, all of which must be answered i.e. 9 minutes per question. Tackle every point raised without being side-tracked. As time is limited it is acceptable to structure your answers in note form or as lists. Don't be tempted to spend more than the allotted time on a topic you know well, as few marks will be gained and much needed thinking time will be lost for weaker areas.

Case Commentaries
There are two case commentaries; both should be answered, ideally spending 45 minutes on each. Answer the question literally; if they ask you to "List the causes of..." then do just that; if you are asked to "Discuss..." you should try to use full sentences, although note form is acceptable if time is a factor.

Usually a brief outline is provided of a common condition found in Primary Care, followed by four or five questions, often interjected with new information as the story unfolds. However, always answer the question at the stage it is posed without the influence of forthcoming information.

Although knowledge of medical management is important, the focus is more on the psychosocial aspects of care of the child and his/her family. It is essential to be familiar with the roles of each member of the Multi-disciplinary team and be able to advise on Health Education & Prevention etc.

THE CLINICAL EXAMINATION

The Long Case
In the Long Case you have 40 minutes with the patient. Time management is an important skill that can only be gained by frequent practice under exam conditions. Introducing yourself and chatting to the child and parents for a few minutes will be time well spent, as they will be far more friendly and co-operative than if you jump in with frantic questions.

Take a full history including antenatal, immunisations, development and the social situation at home and at school. This is traditionally followed by a full examination, although in a potentially fractious toddler take any opportunity to examine the relevant system while the child is still amenable. Always remember to plot height and weight on the growth chart, check the BP and test the urine.

Give yourself 10 minutes at the end to prepare a summary, a differential diagnosis, and a suitable management plan. If you still have no idea of the diagnosis, ask the parents, they will more than likely tell you and always check with them if there are areas they think are important which you haven't covered. If they are still unforthcoming, remember, knowing the diagnosis is not as important as demonstrating you have tried to find out in a logical manner. You then have 20 minutes with the examiners, only 5–10 minutes will be spent on your presentation, the remainder usually being spent testing your knowledge of related aspects to the case. Present the relevant positive or negative findings only. Keep it brief and interesting. List your differential diagnoses in order of probability and avoid mentioning rare causes unless you're prepared to discuss them. End confidently with your initial management plan and be ready to expand on it.

The Short Cases
This section lasts 30 minutes. At least 10 minutes will be developmental assessments and you should be fluent at performing the distraction hearing test, various means of testing vision and eliciting which milestones the child has reached.

The examiners will want to get through as many cases as possible, however, avoid the temptation to lunge at the relevant bit without first introducing yourself and telling the parents and child what you intend to do, although don't procrastinate either.

Know the features of common syndromes (e.g. Down's, Turner's, neurofibromatosis etc.) and when asked to examine a particular system always stick to 'inspection, palpation, percussion and auscultation' – my examination of 'the heart' ended with the observation of a thoracotomy scar. Always be tactful when presenting your findings of an abnormal looking child and remember to thank them before moving on to the next case.

Again the best way of passing the Short Cases is endless practice. Bring a paediatric stethoscope and although all other necessary equipment should be provided, do bring your own if you're more comfortable using it. Finally, dress smartly without being overbearing; NEVER EVER argue with the examiners and of course – Good Luck!

MULTIPLE CHOICE QUESTIONS – PAPER 1

60 questions: time allowed 2 hours
Indicate your correct answers with a tick in the boxes provided

1.1   Regarding consent

❏ A   a child below 16 years of age may give consent for elective medical treatment

❏ B   if a child below 16 years of age refuses surgery it must not be carried out

❏ C   an unmarried father has both financial and intrinsic rights for his child

❏ D   a divorced couple disagree about the need for an elective tonsillectomy in their child, the mother's opinion prevails

❏ E   if emergency surgery is needed and the parents are unavailable, consent must be obtained from a person such as a teacher who is '*in loco parentis*'

1.2   With regard to autism

❏ A   it affects males and females equally

❏ B   usually develops after three years of age

❏ C   drugs such as tranquillisers have a role in the management of autism

❏ D   children with autism commonly have islands of intact intellectual functioning, the so-called 'idiot savant'

❏ E   a diagnosis of autism can be made if the child has two of the following features:
global impairment of language and communication
impairment of social relationships, especially empathy
ritualistic and compulsive phenomenon

1.3 **An 8-year-old girl presents with staining of her underwear and slight yellow discharge at the introitus with no other signs**

❑ A it is urgent to exclude sexual abuse in the first instance
❑ B vulvovaginitis is the most likely diagnosis
❑ C *Gardnerella vaginalis* is a common infecting organism
❑ D lack of labial fat pads protecting the vaginal orifice and the excess acidity of the prepubertal vagina are increased risk factors for infection
❑ E topical dienestrol cream is a useful treatment

1.4 **Concerning accidental paracetamol overdose in a 3-year-old child**

❑ A if ingestion has been within one hour and the child is alert, vomiting should be induced with oral ipecacuanha
❑ B hepatotoxicity is likely if the 4-hour level is > 100 mg/ml
❑ C i.v. acetylcysteine is not effective at preventing liver damage if given eight hours after ingestion
❑ D oral methionine may be used within ten hours of ingestion
❑ E it may be an indication of family disruption

1.5 **A normal 3-year-old child**

❑ A can recognise three colours
❑ B will use more than 200 words but have greater comprehension
❑ C can give first and last name
❑ D can give definitions of more than 20 words
❑ E comprehends the meaning of cold/tired/hungry

1.6 **Acne**

❑ A affects 90% of teenagers and 25% of infants
❑ B is usually caused by excessive levels of testosterone
❑ C *Propionibacterium acnes* is an anaerobic diphtheroid
❑ D in moderate cases, treatment with erythromycin should continue for at least 6–12 months
❑ E Roaccutane (vitamin A analogue) can be tried by the GP for severe cases resistant to all other therapy

1.7 With regard to blood pressure measurement in children

❏ A it should be a routine part of cardiovascular examination
❏ B the correct cuff size should be approximately 2/3 the length of the upper arm
❏ C the 5th Korotkoff sound is used for diastolic measurement
❏ D raised blood pressure in children < six years is commonly due to primary hypertension
❏ E a diastolic pressure > 90 mmHg before 13 years requires treatment

1.8 Cot death/near miss cot death

❏ A if an infant suffers a cot death but their twin appears in excellent health, the parents may be reassured
❏ B apnoea monitors do not decrease the incidence of cot death
❏ C risk factors include viral infections, prone sleeping position, hypothermia and old PVC mattresses
❏ D parents should be taught to recognise and assess signs of illness in their babies and discouraged from frequent visits to the GP that may result in increased anxiety
❏ E parents who stop smoking, significantly decrease the risk of their child suffering a cot death

1.9 Acute bronchiolitis

❏ A up to 50% of cases are secondary to respiratory syncytial virus
❏ B nasopharyngeal aspirate may be used to the direct detection of virus in secretions by immunofluorescence
❏ C ribavirin is an antiviral agent effective against RSV and should be used as a first-line treatment if RSV infection is confirmed
❏ D Ventolin and theophylline have no effect on bronchiolar obstruction under one year of age
❏ E maternal IgA is protective against RSV

1.10   Concerning late walkers

❏ A   97% of children are walking (more than six steps) by
           18 months, the remaining 3% are 'idiopathic' late walkers
❏ B   93–95% of late walkers have no pathological abnormality
❏ C   'bottom-shuffling' in a late walker is a sinister sign
❏ D   all boys with delayed walking should have a muscle biopsy to
           exclude Duchenne's muscular dystrophy
❏ E   cerebral palsy may present with delayed walking

1.11   Signs of physical abuse include

❏ A   petechial rash over the child's face
❏ B   torn frenulum
❏ C   Mongolian blue spot
❏ D   multiple bruising of various ages over the shins of a 7-year-old
           boy
❏ E   metaphyseal avulsion fractures

1.12   Turner's syndrome

❏ A   affects one in 2500 women
❏ B   has the genotype (XY) however, intrauterine development
           persists as female due to lack of receptors for circulating
           testosterone
❏ C   is associated with Crohn's disease
❏ D   features apparent at birth include web neck, low posterior
           hairline and wide spaced nipples
❏ E   somatotrophin (human growth hormone) is a useful treatment
           for short stature once the epiphyses have fused

1.13   Concerning secretory otitis media (glue ear)

❏ A   it can cause a sensorineural hearing loss
❏ B   it may present as a behavioural problem
❏ C   the primary role of the grommet is to drain the middle ear
           effusion
❏ D   most grommets require surgical removal
❏ E   the majority of affected children will have normal hearing by
           eight years of age

1.14   In Henoch-Schönlein purpura

- ❏ A   a diffuse self-limiting vasculitis often follows a viral infection
- ❏ B   a transient small joint arthritis is typical
- ❏ C   other features include abdominal pain and a purpuric rash, especially affecting buttocks and legs (flexor surface)
- ❏ D   50% of children develop microscopic and 20–30% develop macroscopic haematuria
- ❏ E   there is no treatment of proven value

1.15   With regard to eczema

- ❏ A   in 70% there is a family history of atopy
- ❏ B   it resolves by five years in 80% of children
- ❏ C   it often starts on the face/neck/behind the ears, but favours extensor surfaces in older children
- ❏ D   Chinese herbal therapy is of proven benefit in resistant cases
- ❏ E   breast-feeding or hypoallergenic formula milk decreases the risk and severity in infants with a positive family history of atopy

1.16   In *Haemophilus influenzae B*:

- ❏ A   60% of invasive Hib disease presents as meningitis
- ❏ B   the mortality of Hib meningitis is approximately 20%
- ❏ C   Hib infection is rare before two years of age
- ❏ D   Hib vaccination is contraindicated in HIV-positive individuals
- ❏ E   all infants in the absence of genuine contraindications should be vaccinated at two, three and four months of age

1.17   Molluscum contagiosum

- ❏ A   is a pox RNA virus infection
- ❏ B   typically presents with small pearly umbilicated lesions anywhere on the body
- ❏ C   has a low virulence
- ❏ D   the lesions generally take several months to resolve
- ❏ E   removal by piercing the lesion with a sharpened orange stick dipped in phenol or liquid nitrogen are the treatments of choice

1.18   Pityriasis rosea

❏ A   commonly presents in toddlers and young children
❏ B   is often misdiagnosed as ringworm
❏ C   a generalised rash is followed by a solitary scaly indurated
        'herald patch' 2–3 weeks later
❏ D   the generalised rash may be described as having a Christmas
        tree pattern
❏ E   all antibiotics are of no benefit

1.19   Nappy rash

❏ A   typically involves the flexures when due to irritant dermatitis
❏ B   a red rash with satellite lesions and shallow ulcers is typical of
        candidiasis
❏ C   eczematous nappy rash may be improved by encouraging the
        mother to breast-feed.
❏ D   topical Dermovate cream is the treatment of choice for the
        scaly intertriginous rash of eczema
❏ E   nappy rash due to seborrhoeic dermatitis may be associated
        with cradle cap

**1.20   'Health of the Nation' targets that are relevant to the health
         of children and adolescents include**

❏ A   smoking, alcohol consumption and illegal substance abuse
❏ B   healthy diets and prevention of obesity
❏ C   suicide and deliberate self-harm
❏ D   teenage pregnancy and sexually transmitted diseases
❏ E   accident prevention

1.21   Growth charts

❏ A   children aged 0–1 year should have at least three recordings of
        height and weight
❏ B   all children below the second centile for height should be
        reviewed by the GP
❏ C   all children below the first centile for height should be referred
        for a specialist opinion
❏ D   normal growth velocity of children over two years of age is
        10 cm/year
❏ E   children with a growth velocity less than the 25th or greater
        than the 75th centile should be referred for a specialist opinion

1.22   School refusal

❏   A   is most common in children aged 11–14 years
❏   B   children typically come from social class I–II
❏   C   is more common in girls
❏   D   commonly presents with recurrent abdominal pains or headaches
❏   E   typically occurs in a conscientious and intelligent student

1.23   Signs of child abuse include

❏   A   'frozen watchfulness'
❏   B   acute hyphaema
❏   C   a single green/yellow bruise over the forehead of a toddler
❏   D   a midclavicular fracture in a 10-day-old infant
❏   E   scalds over both buttocks

1.24   Munchausen's syndrome by proxy

❏   A   has a mortality of 2–10%
❏   B   confrontation with evidence should be avoided
❏   C   never involves the father
❏   D   may show evidence of failure to thrive
❏   E   generally occurs in pre-school children

1.25   With regard to dermatophyte (ringworm) infections in children

❏   A   tinea pedis is rare in children under five years
❏   B   Trichophyton often causes tinea capitis
❏   C   tinea corporis typically presents with hair loss, circular patches of alopecia with scaling skin and broken hairs
❏   D   are caused by superficial filamentous (hyphae) fungal infections of skin which fluoresce under Wood's light
❏   E   large infected areas may require a two-week course of oral griseofulvin

1.26   Causes of persistent snoring in children include

❏   A   hypertrophic nasal turbinates
❏   B   hyperthyroidism
❏   C   obesity
❏   D   Down's syndrome
❏   E   recurrent tonsillitis

1.27   Club foot

❏   A   is more common in boys
❏   B   the feet are held in equinovalgus
❏   C   may be associated with spina bifida
❏   D   will need surgical repair
❏   E   treatment should be commenced at three months

1.28   Risk factors for congenital dislocation of the hip (CDH) include

❏   A   male sex
❏   B   oligohydramnios
❏   C   sister had CDH
❏   D   forceps delivery
❏   E   maternal drug abuse

1.29   Features of neurofibromatosis include

❏   A   café au lait spots
❏   B   petechial rash
❏   C   duodenal carcinoids
❏   D   hamartomata
❏   E   mental retardation and epilepsy

1.30   A strawberry patch

❏   A   is a congenital cavernous haemangioma
❏   B   90% have completely resolved by three years
❏   C   may cause a generalised petechial rash
❏   D   may calcify
❏   E   when treated with cryotherapy, generally needs several
            sessions before complete resolution is achieved

1.31   Cleft lip

❑   A   has an equal incidence in boys and girls
❑   B   is increasing in incidence
❑   C   affects approximately 1 in 750 live births
❑   D   is associated with cleft palate in less than 20% of cases
❑   E   the risk to a child whose sibling has a cleft lip is 5%

1.32   Signs of severe acute asthma include

❑   A   a normal pCO_2 on an arterial blood gas
❑   B   agitation
❑   C   the use of accessory muscles
❑   D   the presence of pectus carinatum
❑   E   pulsus paradoxus of 10–20 mmHg

1.33   Inguinal hernia in children

❑   A   rarely requires surgical repair
❑   B   generally presents with strangulation
❑   C   should be repaired before one year of age
❑   D   a significant proportion of inguinal herniae become irreducible
            before three months of age
❑   E   may contain an ovary

1.34   Congenital hypertrophic pyloric stenosis

❑   A   has an incidence of 4 per 1000 live births
❑   B   typically presents with projectile bilestained vomiting
❑   C   is more common in girls
❑   D   may cause hyperkalaemic alkalosis
❑   E   investigation of choice is an ultrasound scan

1.35   Tonsillectomy

❑   A   is indicated in children having two attacks of tonsillitis a year
❑   B   complications include development of a quinsy
❑   C   should be performed if parents request a prophylactic
            procedure
❑   D   complications include complete dysphagia
❑   E   post-op secondary haemorrhage is treated with antibiotics

1.36   Mesenteric adenitis

❑   A   often precedes an upper respiratory tract infection (URTI)
❑   B   may give signs of peritonitis
❑   C   is caused by an adenovirus
❑   D   is not typically associated with a fever
❑   E   is associated with a lymphocytosis

1.37   With regard to oesophageal atresia

❑   A   85% of affected babies will have a tracheo-oesophageal fistula
❑   B   it may be associated with cardiovascular and urogenital anomalies
❑   C   mothers often have oligohydramnios antenatally
❑   D   it can present with recurrent pneumonia
❑   E   it is diagnosed by a barium swallow

1.38   Intussusception

❑   A   usually presents between five and 12 months
❑   B   diagnosis is confirmed by USS or barium swallow, which may be therapeutic
❑   C   presents with constant inconsolable crying and drawing up of the legs ± passage of blood PR ('red-currant jelly')
❑   D   may be associated with a viral illness
❑   E   is commonly ileocolic in origin

1.39   Wilms' nephroblastoma

❑   A   commonly presents before five years of age
❑   B   is frequently bilateral
❑   C   often presents with haematuria
❑   D   diagnosis should be confirmed by renal biopsy
❑   E   is the commonest intra-abdominal tumour of childhood

1.40   Acute epiglottitis

❑   A   commonly occurs in infants less than one year of age
❑   B   its incidence has significantly decreased since the introduction of the Hib vaccine
❑   C   is associated with septicaemia
❑   D   the child characteristically holds his head in hyperflexion
❑   E   should be confirmed by a lateral neck X-ray

1.41   Undescended testis

- ❏ A   is present in 15–30% of term male infants
- ❏ B   when present is usually bilateral
- ❏ C   is most commonly found at the superficial inguinal pouch
- ❏ D   orchidopexy should be performed before four years of age
- ❏ E   has an increased incidence of torsion

1.42   Features of cardiac failure include

- ❏ A   tachycardia
- ❏ B   tachypnoea
- ❏ C   sweating
- ❏ D   a gallop rhythm
- ❏ E   excessive weight gain

1.43   With regard to reflexes

- ❏ A   the Moro reflex persists from birth to about four months
- ❏ B   the rooting/suckling and swallowing reflex is usually absent before 34/40
- ❏ C   an absent red reflex may indicate a retinoblastoma
- ❏ D   the grasping reflex persists from birth to about three months
- ❏ E   the stepping reflex persists from birth to about six months

1.44   At six weeks a child

- ❏ A   can support its head when pulled to a sitting position
- ❏ B   can follow a dangling object through a 90° arc
- ❏ C   smiles at familiar faces
- ❏ D   will have developed the parachute reflex
- ❏ E   will have developed the asymmetric tonic neck reflex

1.45   An 8-month-old child

- ❏ A   can roll from the prone to supine position, but can rarely roll back to prone
- ❏ B   can stand while holding on to furniture
- ❏ C   will look for 'lost' objects
- ❏ D   will no longer investigate all objects by 'mouthing'
- ❏ E   should have three or four words that are used in the correct context

1.46   A normal 18-month-old child

❑   A   can balance on one foot for a second
❑   B   can kick a ball forward
❑   C   can walk upstairs holding on, one foot per step
❑   D   can walk backwards
❑   E   may not be walking if a 'bottom-shuffler'

1.47   Known side-effects of sodium valproate include

❑   A   pancreatitis
❑   B   Stevens–Johnson syndrome typically
❑   C   hyperactivity commonly
❑   D   increased appetite and obesity
❑   E   epigastric pain and nausea

1.48   An acute asthma attack may be triggered by

❑   A   exercise
❑   B   gastro-oesophageal reflux
❑   C   climatic change
❑   D   rhinovirus infection
❑   E   emotion

1.49   A normal 3-year-old child

❑   A   can stand on one leg for up to five seconds
❑   B   can walk backwards toe-to-heel
❑   C   usually climb stairs two feet per step
❑   D   will have developed hand dominance
❑   E   can run in a straight line with a narrow stable gait

1.50   Known side-effects of phenytoin include

❑   A   megaloblastic anaemia
❑   B   lymphoma
❑   C   choreoathetosis
❑   D   SLE
❑   E   gum hypertrophy

1.51 The differential diagnoses of asthma include

- ❑ A   inhaled foreign body
- ❑ B   cardiac failure
- ❑ C   cystic fibrosis
- ❑ D   mediastinal lymphadenopathy
- ❑ E   a nervous 'tic'

1.52 Tics

- ❑ A   are defined as stereotypic, repetitive, voluntary movements
- ❑ B   simple developmental tics affect 15% of primary school children
- ❑ C   are generally not of pathological significance and are usually outgrown by four years
- ❑ D   may be manifestations of tension or emotional disorder when they commonly persist beyond adolescence
- ❑ E   may be familial

1.53 Regarding immunisations

- ❑ A   the BCG vaccine is given to infants from high-risk groups only
- ❑ B   the primary course of DPT, Hib & polio comprises three doses given at two, three and four months
- ❑ C   the MMR is ideally given at two years of age
- ❑ D   a booster dose of DT and Hib is given at 3–5 years
- ❑ E   all school-leavers should be given the BCG vaccine

1.54 Treatment of cystic fibrosis includes

- ❑ A   regular physiotherapy
- ❑ B   heart and lung transplant
- ❑ C   long-term prophylactic amoxycillin
- ❑ D   a high protein, low fat diet
- ❑ E   pancreatic enzyme supplements with main meals only

1.55   Childhood asthma

❑ A dehydration is common in asthma, so i.v. fluids should be
        increased to one-third above normal maintenance in severe
        cases
❑ B a CXR on admission should be taken in all children presenting
        with an acute exacerbation
❑ C peak expiratory flow rates (PEFR) should be measured in
        children older than five years
❑ D the commonest reason for a child to be admitted to hospital in
        the UK is for an acute exacerbation of asthma
❑ E i.v. steroids are first-line treatment in all cases of acute
        exacerbation of asthma

1.56   The MMR vaccine

❑ A is contraindicated in patients allergic to neomycin
❑ B should not be given within three weeks of another live vaccine
        (except OPV(Sabin))
❑ C is safe in pregnancy
❑ D commonly results in a rash +/- fever from day 5–10 lasting
        approximately two days
❑ E is contraindicated in patients who have received an injection
        of immunoglobulin within three months

1.57   Contraindications to the MMR vaccination

❑ A presence of fever at the time of vaccination
❑ B HIV infection
❑ C AIDS
❑ D asthma requiring regular twice daily steroid inhalers
❑ E a past medical history of seizures or febrile convulsions

1.58   Pertussis immunisation

❑ A has a definite associated risk of serious brain damage in
        approximately 0.001% of vaccinated children
❑ B is contraindicated with fever of > 39.5°C within 48 hours of a
        previous vaccination
❑ C is contraindicated in children with cerebral palsy
❑ D is contraindicated in children with idiopathic epilepsy
❑ E may result in an increased incidence of febrile convulsions in
        children older than six months

1.59 Concerning immunisations

❑ A polio is transmitted via pharyngeal secretions only
❑ B OPV (Sabin) is contraindicated in children who have immunocompromised siblings
❑ C IPV (Salk) is safe to use in immunocompromised children
❑ D 100% coverage with tetanus vaccination will never result in eradication of this disease
❑ E tetanus toxin boosters should be given every five years

1.60 Bacillus Calmette-Guérin (BCG)

❑ A high-risk infants should have a positive Heaf test before vaccination proceeds
❑ B is safe in asymptomatic HIV-positive patients
❑ C may be given at the same time as other live vaccines
❑ D should be given after a positive tuberculin test
❑ E offers some protection against leprosy

SHORT NOTE QUESTIONS – PAPER 1

10 questions: time allowed 1 hour 30 minutes
Write short notes of the following subjects. Conciseness will be
beneficial. Lists are acceptable.

1. Outline your management of a six-year-old girl presenting with nocturnal enuresis.

2a. Describe the benefits of breast-feeding over bottle feeding.
2b. Outline maternal excretion of drugs in breast milk and list those which are an absolute contra-indication to breast-feeding.

3. Describe the different types of dehydration. Outline your pre-hospital management of a dehydrated infant.

4. Outline methods that may help to lessen the risk of Sudden Infant Death Syndrome.

5a. Describe methods of testing hearing in neonates.
5b. List risk factors for deafness in newborns.

6. Advise a father how to help his children cope with the impending death of their terminally ill mother.

7. Outline your management of a two-month-old infant with a head circumference on the 97th centile.

8a. List the common causes of faecal soiling in a 5-year-old boy.
8b. Discuss your management of this problem.

9. Outline your management of a three-year-old boy whose withdrawn behaviour at play school is causing his teachers concern.

10a. Outline your management of a two-week-old boy whose Guthrie tests have shown a TSH > 100 mu/L.
10b. Discuss your initial counselling of the parents.

CASE COMMENTARIES – PAPER 1

Two questions: time allowed 1 hour 30 minutes
Read the following case history carefully. Then answer <u>all</u> the
questions below. Please start your answer on a separate page.

CASE COMMENTARY 1

Simon is the first child of a banker and his wife. There were no antenatal problems and he was born at 39 weeks after a normal delivery. His postnatal check was unremarkable and he went home at 48 hours.

At a routine visit two weeks later the health visitor is concerned that Simon appears floppy, is not feeding well and seems to have some features suggestive of Down's syndrome.

1.   As their GP how would you respond to this information?

Down's syndrome is subsequently confirmed

2.   How would you counsel the parents at this time?

The parents accept the situation and take good care of Simon, however the father becomes increasingly angry and resentful over the delayed diagnosis and is concerned about the toll it will take on his wife. She has had to give up work and although he works overtime they are still under some financial strain. He feels Simon should go into care and convinces his wife it is for the best.

3.   How might you help them at this point?

CASE COMMENTARY 2

Karl is a 13-year-old boy whose teachers have noticed a marked deterioration over the past five months in his schoolwork from a previous high standard. He has also become unkept, moody, stays out late and is being rude and aggressive to his parents. They have asked you as his GP to see him, but Karl denies there is a problem and insists his parents are overreacting.

1.   **What are the possible explanations behind Karl's change of behaviour and how would you initially manage this problem?**

2.   **What would you discuss with the family at this point?**

Karl's behaviour deteriorates further, his parents find a bottle of dry cleaning fluid under his bed and soon after, he is caught breaking into a car.

3.   **What are the perils to which Karl is being exposed?**

4.   **What is your specific management of this problem and what other professional help may be required?**

5.   **What are the prospects for Karl and his family?**

MULTIPLE CHOICE QUESTION PAPER 1 – ANSWERS

1.1   **Answer: A**

Below 16 years of age, consent of a parent or guardian is required, unless emergency treatment is required (when consent from a person '*in loco parentis*' is also unnecessary) or the child has given consent and the doctor considers that the child is of sufficient understanding to make an informed decision about medical care (including oral contraception) and the child refuses that the parents be asked.

If a child below 16 years of age refuses surgery it can still be carried out if the doctor believes the child doesn't have sufficient understanding to make an informed decision or if a court has considered the child's objection and told the doctor to proceed.

A mother and father have equal parental responsibilities for their legitimate child. If parents disagree it is probably inappropriate to proceed, although only one parent is needed for consent. An unmarried father is only financially responsible for his child, he has no intrinsic rights.

1.2   **Answer: C**

Seventy five per cent of children with autism are male and it usually develops before three years of age. Typical features of autism include: global impairment of language and communication; impairment of social relationships, especially empathy; and ritualistic and compulsive phenomena. All three features should be present before making the diagnosis. The 'idiot savant' is a rare feature of autism, the majority of children have a decreased IQ.

Treatment includes: educational and behavioural modification programmes; parental support and guidance; drugs such as tranquillisers may be needed to control panic attacks and sleep disorders, whereas haloperidol may be used to reduce stereotypes. Finally, residential placement may be necessary in severe cases where families are unable to cope, indeed up to 60% need long-term hospital or institutional care.

1.3   **Answers: B C E**

Vulvovaginitis is the commonest gynaecological disorder in children. Commonly isolated organisms include Gardnerella, bacteroides and Streptococci in pre-pubertal girls. Threadworms may also cause symptoms and a vaginal foreign body should be considered if the discharge is bloodstained or offensive. Risk factors of infection include the lack of labial fat pads protecting the vaginal orifice and lack of the protective acid secretions found during the reproductive years.

Treatment includes: antibiotics if a specific organism is present; excluding an underlying cause e.g. recent broad spectrum antibiotics; attention to vulval hygiene and avoidance of irritants and topical dienestrol cream in refractory cases which may help to clear infection by improving acidity.

If the symptoms are not persistent and in the absence of any other physical or behavioural signs it is wiser not to discuss the possibility of sexual abuse with the mother, unless she expresses concern.

1.4   **Answers: D E**

Inducing vomiting with ipecacuanha and gastric lavage have both fallen out of favour due to, for example the risk of aspiration/oesophageal trauma. Activated charcoal to prevent absorption of paracetamol in the stomach is more commonly used. Hepatotoxicity is likely if the 4-hour level is > 200 mg/L (nomograms are available in all A&E departments). i.v. acetylcysteine is most effective at preventing liver damage if given within eight hours of ingestion, however later treatment is still worth-while. Oral methionine may be used within ten hours of ingestion although i.v. acetylcysteine is the drug of choice.

An accidental overdose may well be an indication of family disruption and when the child is discharged the GP should arrange follow up to check on safety at home (e.g. drugs/household products locked away or out of reach, check containers are well labelled and medication has child-proof lids).

1.5   **Answers: A B C E**

Normal 3-year-old children can recognise three colours, know their full name and will use over 200 words in conversation. However, they can only define about six words from around 3–4 years, but will comprehend the meaning of various sensations, such as cold/tired/hungry.

1.6   **Answers: A C D**

Acne affects 90% of teenagers and 25% of infants. Boys are more commonly affected than girls and it persists beyond the age of 25 in 15%. Acne is usually associated with normal levels of testosterone. Causes include medication (e.g. oral contraceptive pill, steroids, phenytoin), irritants (e.g. cosmetics), occlusion (e.g. friction by head bands), emotional stress, menstruation and endocrine abnormalities (e.g. Cushing's, diabetes, virilizing tumour, polycystic ovaries).

Propionibacterium acnes is an anaerobic diphtheroid and this together with yeast colonises the blocked sebaceous glands and breaks down sebum releasing free fatty acids which cause an inflammatory reaction in the dermis. Secondary infection of papules cause pustules, cysts and scars.

In moderate cases, the treatment with erythromycin should continue for at least 6–12 months as its maximum effect is not achieved before 3–6 months. Even so, it may still relapse requiring a further three months treatment, thus the patient must be well motivated. Severe cases (multiple cysts, pits, scars and keloids) and resistant moderate cases should be referred to the dermatologist. Roaccutane should only be prescribed by the hospital specialist. Liver function tests and lipids should be checked before starting and monitored throughout. It causes dry skin and mucosa and is 100% teratogenic (therefore oral contraception should be continued for at least one month after cessation of treatment).

1.7   **Answers: B E**

Routine blood pressure measurement in children is not part of a screening test but should be measured during the cardiovascular examination if indicated (i.e. in the presence of a cardiac murmur, history of renal/endocrine disease, malignant hypertension and family history (e.g. phaeochromocytoma) or if there are signs of malignant hypertension (e.g. papilloedema), renal or adrenal masses, renal artery bruit, goitre, radio-femoral delay and neurofibromatosis found on examination).

The correct cuff size should be approximately 2/3 the length of the upper arm. The 5th Korotkoff sound is often not heard in childhood, therefore K4 is used until adolescence when K5 is used. In infants it is easier to use ultrasound doppler or more typically 'Dinamopp'. Results can be checked against a graph of normal values for age.

Secondary hypertension is commoner in younger children and higher blood pressures. After 13 years 50% is due to primary hypertension and 50% is due to secondary hypertension (of which 80% is renal parenchymal disease, 10% renal vascular disease and 10% 'other').

The level of hypertension requiring treatment is not really known but most clinicians treat a diastolic blood pressure > 90 before 13 years and > 100 after 13 years. N.B. Three or so recordings should be taken some weeks apart (in general) before a diagnosis of hypertension is made.

1.8   **Answers: B E**

If an infant suffers a cot death it is important to ensure the health of all siblings, especially twins who are at increased risk and should always be admitted for observation, full septic screen and possible investigations for inherited metabolic disorders. Other risk factors include viral infections, hyperthermia (from over wrapping/prone sleeping position), old PVC mattresses and parental smoking, indeed parents who stop smoking have been shown to significantly decrease the risk of their child suffering a cot death.

Apnoea monitors do not decrease the incidence of cot death and their use is controversial. Advantages include their reassurance, ease of use and portability. However they are expensive and often leads to false alarms leading to increased anxiety. They do not detect hypoxia and transcutaneous oxygen monitoring is under evaluation as an alternative. All parents issued with an alarm must be trained in basic life support.

Parents should be taught to recognise and assess signs of illness in their babies and a system of increased surveillance by health visitors and GP should be instated. Parents should be encouraged to consult their GP more readily and should not be criticised for it.

1.9 **Answers: B D**

More than 70% of acute bronchiolitis is due to RSV, the rest is secondary to adenovirus, rhinovirus, parainfluenza 1, 2 & 3 and influenza A. Nasopharyngeal aspirate leads to the detection of virus in secretions by immunofluorescence. Ribavirin is an antiviral agent effective against RSV, however it is very expensive and therefore treatment should probably be reserved for 'high risk' babies (e.g. prems, broncho-pulmonary dysplasia, congenital heart disease); the severely ill ($pO_2 <$ 8.6 or increased pCO_2) or infants less than six weeks old.

Ventolin and theophylline have no effect on bronchiolitic obstruction in those under one year and there is limited evidence that Atrovent is beneficial. Maternal IgG is protective against RSV.

1.10 **Answers: A B E**

Ninety seven per cent of children are walking (more than six steps) by 18 months, the remaining 3% are 'idiopathic' late walkers. 93–95% of late walkers have no pathological abnormality, features of which include a family history (especially 'bottom-shuffling'), hypotonia (especially legs), late sitting, lax joints (back-kneeing/poor leg bulk) and non weight bearing. All boys with delayed walking should have a full neurological examination by a paediatrician and consideration of investigations including a serum CPK to exclude Duchenne's muscular dystrophy followed by an EMG and muscle biopsy if this is elevated. Mild/moderate spastic diplegia may present as late walking. The diagnosis is indicated in children with hypertonia (except 'bottom-shufflers'), brisk reflexes and difficulty in dorsiflexion of their feet.

1.11 **Answers: A B E**

A facial petechial rash maybe a sign of smothering, although it may also be present in whooping cough. A generalised petechial rash however, should raise suspicion of idiopathic thrombocytopenic purpura or meningococcal septicaemia. Multiple bruising over the shins of a seven-year-old boy is a normal finding, but bruising in a child less than nine months over the face, upper arms, wrists or inner thighs (+/- grip marks) must cause concern. A Mongolian blue spot is commonly mistaken for abuse, but is in fact a harmless congenital blue marking, frequently occurring over the buttocks and sacrum.

Other superficial features of physical child abuse include bite marks, a torn frenulum (from, for example, forced bottle feeding), lacerations, ligature marks, burns and scalds.

Bony injuries include metaphyseal or epiphyseal fractures, which are suspicious of a twisting or pulling injury. Also, multiple fractures at different stages of healing or delayed presentation of fractures need very careful assessment.

1.12   **Answers: A C D**

Turner's syndrome affects 1 in 2500 women. It has the genotype (XO) and mosaicism may occur with the genotype (XO, XX). N.B. testicular feminisation has the genotype (XY).

Features apparent at birth include web neck, low posterior hairline and wide spaced nipples. Other features include 'shield shaped' chest, coarctation of the aorta, left heart defects, cubitus valgus, short stature (less than 130 cm), hyperconvex nails, nystagmus, 'streak' ovaries – rudimentary or absent and an association with Crohn's disease.

Somatotrophin is a useful treatment for short stature but only before the epiphyses have fused. Counselling is also an important part of the treatment and should include genetic, medical and infertility issues.

1.13   **Answers: B E**

Glue ear causes a conductive hearing loss and the resulting deafness may present with behavioural problems due to the child's frustration. The natural history of the condition means that most children will have normal hearing by eight years of age regardless. However, early treatment is vital to ensure that the hearing is adequate for normal development.

Surgical treatment involves myringotomy and insertion of grommets, the latter allows the middle ear to be ventilated – a role that will eventually be resumed by the Eustachian tube. The majority are extruded two months to two years following insertion.

1.14   **Answers: A D E**

Henoch-Schönlein purpura is a diffuse self-limiting vasculitis that usually transiently affects the large joints; the purpuric rash classically affects the buttocks and extensor surfaces of the legs. Abdominal pain often occurs and may be the presenting symptom. Most haematuria resolves spontaneously. Heavy proteinuria may indicate diffuse rapidly progressive glomerulonephritis often with a nephrotic phase. A small number develop severe hypertension and acute renal failure requiring dialysis.

There is no proven treatment although in severely ill patients with life-threatening glomerulonephritis combined treatment with cytotoxins, anticoagulants and corticosteroids has been tried. Follow up should continue for at least three months or until urinary abnormalities have disappeared.

1.15   **Answers: A D E**

Atopic eczema is very common, affecting up to 10% of children and its incidence is increasing. It generally occurs before six months, but can start at any age. 50% of cases have resolved by five years and 80% by ten years. It may occur anywhere, but favours flexural surfaces in older children.

Initial treatment includes preventative measures such as avoidance of irritants and feeding high-risk infants with breast or hypoallergenic formula milks. Breast-feeding mothers should also avoid consuming common food allergens (e.g. cows' milk or eggs). Other more active treatment methods include skin emollients, topical steroids and antibiotics for secondary infection. Chinese herbal treatment has been shown to be effective, although its mechanism is unknown and periodic cases of liver damage are well documented.

1.16   **Answers: A E**

Hib infection is rare before three months, the incidence then steadily rises to a peak at approximately 10–11 months and then declines to the age of four years. All children less than 13 months should therefore receive the full vaccination course. From 13 months to two years un-immunised children should receive a single Hib dose with their MMR (children are less at risk in this age group and therefore a single dose is effective). The Hib vaccine is not live and is therefore safe in immunocompromised patients.

Sixty per cent of invasive Hib disease presents as meningitis, 15% presents as epiglottitis, 10% presents as septicaemia alone and the remaining 15% includes septic arthritis, osteomyelitis, cellulitis, pneumonia and pericarditis. It has a mortality rate of approximately 2%.

1.17   **Answers: B D**

Molluscum contagiosum is a pox DNA virus infection that typically presents as small pearly umbilicated lesions anywhere on the body with characteristic satellite spread around the original lesion. The incubation period is 2–7 weeks spreading easily to siblings (e.g. via bath water) and the child remains infectious as long as the lesions are present. Atopic and immunocompromised children are particularly susceptible. The treatment of choice is patience as spontaneous resolution is the rule, typically after several months. Removal with phenol or liquid nitrogen is generally reserved for cosmetic reasons only.

1.18   **Answers: B D E**

Pityriasis rosea is probably due to a virus and generally affects adolescents and young adults with a peak incidence in the spring or autumn. The 'herald patch' is a 1–5 cm scaly indurated lesion that precedes the main eruption by 2–3 weeks and is often mistaken for ringworm.

The generalised rash is slightly itchy and mainly affects the trunk and limbs proximally. It comprises small red ovoid macules with centripetal scaling inclining downwards in the skin cleavage from the midline (i.e. Christmas tree pattern, especially seen on the back). It is a self-limiting condition lasting approximately six weeks. Treatment is symptomatic only and may include topical emollients and antihistamines.

1.19   **Answers: B C E**

Both irritant and contact dermatitis spare the flexures and should be treated by exposure to fresh air as much as is possible, frequent nappy changes, careful cleansing with baby lotion and routine use of barrier creams (e.g. zinc/castor oil). Secondary infection may be treated initially with a local antiseptic or antimicrobial. Candida presents as a red rash with satellite lesions and shallow ulcers and should be treated with antifungal cream to skin and gel to white oral/mucosal lesions.

Nappy rash secondary to eczema may be improved by encouraging breast-feeding until three months, avoiding common food allergens (e.g. cows' milk or eggs) and non specific irritants (e.g. soap, wool, over-heating). If eczema fails to settle using emollients while bathing and aqueous creams afterwards, then 0.5–1% hydrocortisone may be applied to the face and intertriginous areas. Potent fluorinated steroids (i.e. Dermovate) should only be used on thicker areas for less than 2–4 weeks and only if treatment with mild-moderate steroids has been unsuccessful.

Seborrhoeic dermatitis is an erythematous greasy rash which commonly involves the nappy area, the occipital region and behind the ears. It may become secondarily infected with Candida requiring treatment with antifungals.

1.20   **Answers: A B C D E**

Health promotion is now a major part of health policy in 'Health of the Nation' targets for ischaemic heart disease and stroke, mental illness, HIV and sexual health, cancer and accident prevention. Important areas relating specifically to children and adolescents include smoking, alcohol consumption, illegal substance abuse, healthy diets, obesity, suicide, deliberate self-harm, accidents, teenage pregnancy and sexually transmitted disease.

1.21   **Answers: B E**

Between 0–1 year a child should ideally have at least five recordings of weight and probably one or two recordings of length; between 1–2 years they should have at least three recordings and those over two should be recorded annually. Measurements should be plotted on (New 9) centile charts as part of a screen for growth failure. All children below the second centile should be reviewed by the GP, especially if the child has tall parents. The GP should also review all children crossing a centile, even if still within normal limits or if there is parental concern. All children below the 0.4th centile should be referred for a specialist opinion.

Normal growth velocity of children over two years is 5 cm/year and is calculated by the formula: (increase in height in cm x 12)/number of months = cm/year.

1.22   **Answers: B D E**

Truancy is associated with children over eight years whereas school refusal commonly occurs in children between 5–11 years. They are typically from a small conventional social class I–II family who may collude over their child's non-attendance.

There is an equal incidence between boys and girls (truancy being more common in boys) and it commonly presents with various psychosomatic features.

1.23   **Answers: A B E**

If a child has an unkempt, frightened withdrawn appearance with 'frozen watchfulness' and possibly, failure to thrive, developmental delay and evidence of physical injury then practitioners should have a high degree of suspicion of abuse.

An acute hyphaema (i.e. blood in the anterior chamber of the eye) may result from serious shaking and scalds over both buttocks are typical of a forced immersion. However, a midclavicular fracture in a 10-day-old infant may have resulted from a difficult delivery and although a green/yellow bruise is evidence of an old injury (more precise estimation from the colour of the bruise is notoriously unreliable), this is a common finding in an active toddler.

1.24   **Answers: A D E**
Munchausen's by proxy refers to signs or symptoms in a child deliberately fabricated or induced by an adult. The child may be normal or have an illness and is usually pre-school. Although no organic cause can be found for the symptoms and all investigations are normal, the child may well show evidence of emotional abuse and/or failure to thrive. It is associated with a mortality of 2–10%. The perpetrator is usually the mother, rarely the father, often with some kind of medical knowledge or training (e.g. nurse). She is generally not psychiatrically unwell, but often has a personality disorder with maladaptation in other areas. She may have been abused herself as a child and is now seeking the attention of carers or she may be seeking refuge from other problems. Confrontation with evidence, while involving the partner is a key part of the management. This should be done in a sympathetic manner. A case conference should be organised to consider the child's welfare, who should ideally stay with the family if at all possible. Further help should be offered in the form of counselling, psychiatric referral and family/behavioural therapy.

1.25   **Answers: A B**
Tinea pedis (athlete's foot) is common in adolescents, leading to itchy, macerated and peeling skin between the toes with an unpleasant odour. Tinea capitis (scalp ringworm) is often caused by Trichophyton and results in hair loss, circular patches of alopecia with scaling skin and broken hairs. Tinea corporis results in itching ± scaly circular lesions anywhere on the skin. There may also be small vesicles at the periphery. The differential diagnosis includes eczema, psoriasis and the 'Herald patch' of pityriasis rosea. *Microsporum canis* infections fluoresce under Wood's light. Fungal infections are identified by examining skin scrapings and plucked hairs under the microscope for hyphae and spores.
Small areas may be treated with topical clotrimazole cream, however large areas require a 4–6 week course of oral griseofulvin. The rest of the family (including pets) should be examined and treated as necessary.

1.26   **Answers: A C D E**
Causes of persistent snoring include hypertrophic nasal turbinates, allergic rhinitis, deviated nasal septum, nasal polyps, obesity and hypothyroidism. Recurrent tonsillitis may result in permanently enlarged tonsils which predisposes to persistent snoring as does the macroglossia associated with Down's syndrome.

1.27   Answers: A C

There is a male to female ratio of 2:1. The feet are held in equinovarus (i.e. downwards and inward) and it is associated with spina bifida. Initial management begins within one week of birth with splintage, where the deformity is 'overcorrected'. The infant then has weekly foot manipulations and if the foot has not corrected by approximately three months operative reduction or tendon release and fixation may be necessary.

1.28   Answers: B C

Unstable hips are found in 1% of hips at birth and are more common on the left (60%). Risk factors include female sex (80%), family history, breech delivery, first child and history of oligohydramnios. Screening involves the Ortolani-Barlow manoeuvre with USS of suspicious joints (X-rays are unhelpful before six weeks). If these tests are positive, neonates should be splinted in abduction for 6–12 weeks with clinical and radiological follow-up at three, six and twelve months. Most hips will have stabilised with conservative methods however, those with persistent instability will need surgery. This is more likely if initial treatment was delayed.

1.29   Answers: A C E

Dermatological manifestations of neurofibromatosis include multiple fleshy skin nodules (neurofibromas), axillary freckling and more than five café au lait spots, which may be large (1–20 cm), irregular, light brown and occur mainly on the torso. Mental retardation and epilepsy occur in 10% of patients due to diffuse cortical dysgenesis.

1.30   Answers: A C D E

A strawberry patch is a congenital cavernous haemangioma which usually appears a few weeks after birth, growing rapidly in the first few months reaching a maximum by about one year of age and resolving spontaneously before ten years. They may calcify, ulcerate and bleed and if large may cause thrombocytopenia secondary to sequestration. Treatment is usually only necessary if the haemangioma interferes with vital structures (e.g. an eyelid lesion obstructing vision).

1.31   Answers: B C E

Cleft palate has an equal (and increasing) incidence between boys and girls. Cleft lip is more common in boys and affects 1 in 750 live births and is associated with cleft palate in approximately 50% of cases. The risk to a child with one affected sibling is 5% and is 9% with two affected siblings.

1.32   **Answers: A B C**

A normal arterial pCO_2 is an ominous sign, as a patient with acute asthma usually hyperventilates and consequently has a low arterial pCO_2. A normal pCO_2 implies the patient is becoming exhausted and beginning to hypoventilate and may indicate impending respiratory arrest as the pCO_2 continues to climb.

The British Thoracic Society guidelines define acute severe asthma as being: too breathless to talk; too breathless to feed; respirations > 50/min, pulse > 140/min and a PEFR < 50% predicted or best. Other features of life-threatening asthma include a PEFR < 33% predicted or best; a silent chest or poor respiratory effort; agitation, fatigue, decreased level of consciousness and central cyanosis (N.B. Peripheral cyanosis is of little predictive value as it may be affected by numerous causes including the weather!).

Pulsus paradoxus of > 20 mmHg is said to indicate severe acute asthma, although this is a difficult sign to demonstrate and is rarely used. Pectus carinatum, however, is a sign of chronic asthma and has no significance regarding the severity of an acute attack.

1.33   **Answers: C D E**

10% of affected children present with irreducible inguinal hernias, with an increased incidence in the first three months. Prompt elective surgery is essential before one year of age to prevent obstruction and strangulation.

1.34   **Answers: A E**

Pyloric stenosis has an incidence of 4 per 1000 live births with boys being affected more than girls in a ratio of 4:1. Approximately 15% of affected infants have a positive family history, mainly on the mother's side. Vomiting occurs after feeds and becomes projectile but is not bile stained, as the obstruction is so high. Persistent vomiting leads to hyperchloraemic, hypokalaemic alkalosis needing fluid replacement with 0.9% normal saline plus added potassium.

Examination may reveal an olive shaped abdominal mass during a test feed and an USS is the investigation of choice. A barium meal is also useful although may be associated with an increased risk of aspiration. Treatment is surgical by Ramstedt's pyloromyotomy.

1.35   **Answer: E**

Tonsillectomy is indicated in children having more than four attacks of acute tonsillitis per year causing significant systemic illness, interference with growth and school loss or recurrent cervical adenitis or peritonsillar abscess. It has a significant morbidity and mortality and should only be performed if clinically indicated and not at parental request.

Although swallowing is uncomfortable, this does not lead to complete dysphagia post-operatively. Other complications include primary haemorrhage, occurring within 24 hours and usually due to an inadequately ligated/cauterised vessel, and secondary haemorrhage, which is commonly due to infection and occurs in 1% of patients approximately one week following the procedure. Quinsy (peritonsillar abscess) is a complication of tonsillitis and not tonsillectomy.

1.36   **Answers: C E**

Mesenteric adenitis often follows an URTI and is associated with lymphadenopathy elsewhere, especially in the cervical and axillary nodes. It presents with poorly localised, intermittent abdominal pain with no signs of peritonitis and often a high pyrexia (38°C) and lymphocytosis. It may be recurrent. It is frequently caused by an adenovirus and treatment with simple analgesia is sufficient.

1.37   **Answers: A B D**

Eighty five per cent of infants with oesophageal atresia will have a tracheo-oesophageal fistula and 30% will have another abnormality. It may be part of the 'VACTERL' syndrome (i.e. Vertebral, Anorectal, Cardiovascular Tracheo-oesophageal, Renal and Limb anomalies).

It may present with recurrent pneumonia and other signs include cough, airway obstruction (excessive secretions), abdominal distension and cyanotic episodes during feeding. It is diagnosed by the inability to pass a catheter into the stomach, which will be seen on X-ray to be coiled in the oesophagus. Contrast radiology should be avoided due to risk of aspiration. Mothers typically have polyhydramnios antenatally.

1.38   **Answers: A D E**

Intussusception usually presents between five and 12 months, but can occur at any age. Features include intermittent inconsolable crying with drawing up of their legs. Abdominal examination may reveal a 'sausage shaped' mass and the child may pass the classic, but uncommon, 'red currant jelly' stool (a very late sign). Although a definite cause is found in less than 10%, lymphoid hyperplasia in Peyer's patches during a viral illness is thought to be the fulcrum to the principally ileocolic intussusceptions – however any site in the GI tract may be affected. Diagnosis is confirmed by USS or control enema with air or barium which may be therapeutic.

1.39   **Answers: A C E**

Wilms' nephroblastoma is the commonest of all childhood malignant tumours accounting for 10% of cases. It presents before five years of age in 80% of children with a median age of 3.5 years. 95% are unilateral and 20% have metastasised at presentation, mainly to the lung and liver. 80% present with an abdominal mass, 25% with haematuria and approximately 30% with flank pain. Other features include failure to thrive and hemihypertrophy. It may be sporadic or familial, when Wilms' may be associated with aniridia, GU malformations and retardation (WAGR syndrome). The Wilms' tumour gene is found on chromosome 11. Investigations of choice include IVU (renal pelvis distortion, hydro-nephrosis), USS and CT. Renal biopsy should be avoided. Treatment involves nephrectomy, chemotherapy (e.g. actinomycin E) and radio-therapy which can be curative (80% five year survival). It is staged as follows:

Stage I: tumour confined to kidney
Stage II: extrarenal spread but resectable
Stage III: extensive abdominal disease
Stage IV: distant metastases
Stage V: bilateral disease

1.40   **Answers: B C**
Acute epiglottitis is caused by *Haemophilus influenzae* type B. It generally occurs between two to six years of age and the diagnosis is made from the history and classic clinical appearance. Within a few hours of developing a sore throat the child becomes hot, toxic, drooling due to difficulty swallowing, unable to speak and is anxious. The child is dyspnoeic, has inspiratory stridor, subcostal recession and typically holds his head in hyperextension to keep the airway clear and there is usually no cough. Anything that may increase the child's distress should be avoided as this may precipitate a respiratory arrest requiring an emergency attempt at endotracheal intubation by junior staff. This includes unnecessary investigations, such as a lateral neck X-ray and examination of the throat is absolutely contraindicated. If the condition is suspected an experienced anaesthetist should called to perform an elective endotracheal intubation in a controlled environment, such as theatre.

1.41   **Answers: C E**
Undescended testis occurs in 2–3% of term male neonates but in 15–30% of premature babies. Only 25% of cases are bilateral. If the testis is truly undescended it will lie anywhere along the path of descent from the abdominal cavity. Other sites include the perineum, femoral region or base of penis. Orchidopexy must be performed before two years of age to preserve function, preferably at one year. There is an increased incidence of torsion and also neoplasia (e.g. seminoma) which still persists despite surgery.

1.42   **Answers: A B C D E**

1.43   **Answers: A B C D**
The stepping reflex persists to six weeks only.

1.44   **Answers: C E**
When an infant is placed in the supine position his arm will extend in the direction he is looking while the opposite arm will be flexed, this is known as the asymmetric tonic neck reflex which develops at birth and persists until about five months. A six-week-old child can also follow a dangling object through a 45° arc and recognises his main carers (e.g. mother). Head control does not develop until 4–5 months and the parachute reflex (which involves thrusting his arms forward for protection when swooped downwards headfirst) does not develop until 6–9 months.

1.45   **Answers: B C**

An eight-month-old child should be able to roll from prone to supine to prone and most should be able to pull themselves to a standing position with a minority being able to walk while holding onto furniture. Their concept of 'permanence' has developed and they will look for 'lost' objects. Investigation of objects by 'mouthing' begins at around six months and persists until about one year of age. They will have developed non-specific two syllable babble by eight months (e.g. mama/dada) and may copy sounds but use of three or four words in the correct context does not develop until around a year to 18 months.

1.46   **Answers: A D E**

A normal 18-month-old child can kick a ball forward, this develops between 15 months and two years. They can walk backwards from about one year and can climb upstairs holding on, but use two feet per step. They cannot balance on one foot as this develops later at around 22 months to three years. 'Bottom-shufflers' may be delayed walkers although most children walk well by 14 months.

1.47   **Answer: A D E**

Common side-effects of sodium valproate include gastric irritation, nausea, ataxia and tremor, hyperammonaemia, increased appetite and weight gain and transient hair loss (regrowth may be curly). Also impaired liver function and rarely pancreatitis. Stevens–Johnson syndrome is typical of phenytoin and hyperactivity is usually associated with clonazepam and phenobarbitone – sodium valproate being more commonly linked with drowsiness.

1.48   **Answers: A B C D E**

Infection with the parainfluenzae and rhinovirus are viruses particularly likely to precipitate an acute asthma attack.

1.49   **Answers: A D E**

A normal 3-year-old child can stand on one leg for up to five seconds, run in a straight line and should have developed the adult pattern of climbing stairs, one foot per step. Hand dominance is present, but they should not be able to walk backwards toe-to-heel as this generally develops around the age of four.

1.50   **Answers: A B C D E**

Common side-effects of phenytoin include nausea, vomiting, mental confusion, dizziness, headache and tremor. Coarse facies, acne, hirsutism and gingival hyperplasia are particularly undesirable in adolescent patients. Rarer side-effects include dyskinesias, SLE, erythema multiforme (Stevens–Johnson syndrome) and blood disorders. Plasma calcium may be lowered (rickets and osteomalacia). Ataxia, slurred speech, nystagmus and blurred vision are signs of overdosage.

1.51   **Answers: A B C D E**

Any obstructive lesion of the trachea or bronchus (i.e. mediastinal lymphadenopathy) will result in wheeze, as will cardiac failure, which may be suggested by cardiomegaly seen on the chest X-ray. N.B. Asthma causes signs throughout the chest, while some of these lesions produce focal signs.

1.52   **Answers: B C E**

Tics are defined as stereotypic, repetitive, involuntary movements. Simple developmental tics affect 15% of primary school children. They involve movements of the head, neck and shoulders (e.g. blinking, sniffing, shrugging) and are not generally of pathological significance. Most are usually outgrown by four years of age and rarely persist beyond adolescence. Tics may be familial in origin.

1.53   **Answers: A B**

Vaccine	Age	Comment
BCG	Infancy	High risk groups (usually)
DPT Hib Polio	1st dose – 2 months 2nd dose – 3 months 3rd dose – 4 months	Primary course
MMR	12–15 months	Or any time after 12 months if not already given
DT booster Polio booster MMR – 2nd dose	3–5 years	3 years after completion of primary course
BCG	10–14 years	
DT booster Polio booster	13–18 years	

1.54 **Answers: A B**
Treatment of cystic fibrosis includes regular (twice-daily) chest physiotherapy and postural drainage which is essential in preventing and treating chest infections – the parents are usually taught to do this. A small number of children have had successful heart-lung transplants, however donors are always limited and for most chronic patients surgery is not an option because of their poor general condition. Prophylactic flucloxacillin or other antistaphylococcal antibiotics are helpful in avoiding staphylococcal chest infections, although there are conflicting opinions over the efficacy of this policy. Acute infections should be treated with 'best guess' antibiotics until cultures become available.
Patients have high-energy requirements and therefore need a high calorie diet with a normal protein, carbohydrate and high fat content. Fat restriction is no longer recommended as fat is the most energy dense food. Rather supplemental pancreatic enzymes should be taken before all meals and snacks to prevent the clinical features of pancreatic insufficiency (i.e. loose stools and steatorrhoea).

1.55 **Answers: C D**
The commonest reason for a child to be admitted to hospital in the UK is for an acute exacerbation of asthma. Initial investigations should include a PEFR in children older than five years, however it is difficult to measure accurately in younger children and is therefore not a reliable measure of severity in this group. A CXR is not required routinely and is only indicated if the diagnosis is in doubt or an associated severe infection or pneumothorax is clinically suspected. i.v. steroids should only be given with an acute exacerbation if the child is vomiting, otherwise oral preparations are sufficient. i.v. fluids should be restricted to two-thirds of normal maintenance, as increased secretion of antidiuretic hormone occurs with severe asthma resulting in fluid retention.

1.56 **Answers: A B D E**
The MMR vaccine is contraindicated in patients who are allergic to neomycin, kanamycin and those who have had a previous anaphylactic reaction to egg (the vaccine preservative). The MMR vaccine should not be given within three weeks of another live vaccine as this results in a suboptimal response. Likewise, it is contraindicated in patients who have received an injection of immunoglobulin within three months as no response will be mounted in the presence of immunoglobulin that may contain measles, mumps or rubella antibodies.
Pregnancy should be avoided for at least one month after immunisation, which may well result in a rash ± fever from about day 5–10 lasting approximately two days. It is therefore sensible to provide advice on temperature control at the time of vaccination.

1.57   **Answer: A**

The presence of a fever at the time of immunisation is a contraindication for the MMR vaccine. Steroid therapy is a contraindication but only if given in a dose equivalent to prednisolone > 2 mg/kg/day for over one week in the last three months. Neither HIV nor AIDS are contraindicated because MMR produces an antibody response.

1.58   **Answers: B E**

Serious brain damage with the pertussis vaccination occurs extremely rarely, if at all. It has been equivocally implicated in 1 in 2×10^6 immunisations. It may also result in an increased incidence of febrile convulsions in children over six months of age, although not in children less than six months. Other common side-effects include pain and fever and advice should always be given on temperature control.

Contraindications to the pertussis vaccine include; a previous severe reaction, i.e. indurated redness covering most of the arm (or thigh); a fever > 39.5°C within 48 hours of a previous vaccination; or other generalised reaction, including anaphylaxis, prolonged inconsolable screaming or other CNS signs (e.g. seizures) occurring within 72 hours. Those children with stable CNS conditions (e.g. cerebral palsy, spina bifida) particularly benefit from vaccination and most children with idiopathic epilepsy or those with an affected first degree relative should also be immunised. However, an expert opinion must always be sought if in doubt.

1.59   **Answers: B C D**

Polio is transmitted via pharyngeal secretions and via the faeces. OPV (Sabin) results in gut immunity. It is therefore contraindicated in children with immunocompromised siblings as the live vaccine may persist in the child's stool for six weeks afterwards, thus putting their siblings at risk of infection. IPV (Salk) is an inactivated organism and therefore safe to use in the presence of immunodeficiency.

100% coverage with tetanus vaccination will never result in eradication of this disease because tetanus is not spread from person-to-person, but rather via contaminated wounds etc. The 5-dose regime results in immunity lasting at least 10 years, and further boosters are unnecessary before this.

1.60   **Answers: C E**

High-risk infants do not require skin testing before vaccination up to three months of age. The BCG should only be given after a negative tuberculin test. BCG may be given with other live vaccines, otherwise a gap of more than three weeks should be observed between injections or a suboptimal response to both vaccines may ensue. Live OPV which works by inducing gut immunity is the exception and can be given at any time. HIV infection is an absolute contraindication to BCG vaccination.

1.   *Outline your management of a six-year-old girl presenting with nocturnal enuresis.*

ASSESSMENT

History

- Age of child
- Just at night? Primary or secondary? How often? - and if secondary ask regarding stress/urinary symptoms
- Any pattern? (late night stress, birth/bereavement in the family)
- When is bedtime? When does she generally wet the bed?
- How do the parents react? Do they reprimand?
- Is the toilet far from the child's bedroom?
- Any daytime symptoms of urgency/frequency?
- Any family history of bladder/bowel problems?
- What is the child's reaction to wetting?
- Is there a history of constipation?

Examination

- Need to exclude an organic cause
- Do a full examination including blood pressure and neurological examination (bladder S1 root, lower limb neurology, spine, reflexes)
- Height and weight

Investigations

- Urinalysis and MSU for microscopy, culture and sensitivities
- If an organic cause suspected consider renal ultrasound scan
- Further investigations may be indicated if the above are positive e.g. DMSA, DPTA, MAG-3

MANAGEMENT

If the parents are unconcerned and if a child is under 5 years then no management is required. However, as this child is 6 years old she must have regular follow-up and the parents need reassurance that although this is an inconvenient problem, it is not serious and seldom persists beyond childhood. Explain that nocturnal enuresis is a very common problem (10% at 5 years, 5% at 10 years, boys more commonly than girls). A child needs parental support; criticism or intolerance leads to increased anxiety which exacerbates the problem. Reward systems are helpful e.g. star charts (ignore wet nights), as is implementing night time routines, such as last drink at 6 p.m.; voiding at bedtime; and setting the alarm clock to just before the usual time of enuresis to pre-empt any accidents.

The pad and buzzer alarm is useful in older children but needs careful demonstration and regular follow-up. It has a success rate of up to 70%, with children staying dry for longer than 6 weeks, although some relapse.

Medication may be useful for short-term use in older children, such as 'going on holiday' e.g. Desmopressin tablets. It is not as effective as pad and alarm system; however there is improvement of up to 80% within days, but only 12–40% remain completely dry and there is a high relapse rate. Imipramine is not currently recommended.

2a.   *Describe the benefits of breast-feeding over bottle feeding.*

Advantages

- Enjoyable and facilitates bonding
- Is always available, more convenient and 'ready prepared', it is difficult to over feed
- Ideal protein to fat ratio (fore milk has an increased protein content and hind milk an increased fat content)
- More interesting as taste varies with maternal diet
- There is a decreased incidence of eczema in infants of atopic parents
- Provides good (not 100%) contraception via prolactin suppression of ovulation
- Secretory IgA and white cells protect the gut directly from bacterial/viral infection
- Recent studies show that babies may have a higher IQ than those fed on formula milk.

2b. *Outline maternal excretion of drugs in breast milk and list those which are an absolute contra-indication to breast-feeding.*

Most drugs are excreted in breast milk but in amounts that are too small to harm the baby. The amount available for absorption by the infant is generally less than 1–2% of the maternal dose. The milk/plasma ratio for most drugs is between 0.35 and 1.0 varying with the drug pH, dose interval, protein binding and lipid solubility.

Breast-feeding is contra-indicated during maternal treatment with the following drugs:
- Cytotoxins
- Radio-pharmaceuticals
- Lithium
- Ergot alkaloids
- Chloramphenicol

3. *Describe the different types of dehydration. Outline your pre-hospital management of a dehydrated infant.*

There are three types of dehydration:
- Isotonic (water and sodium are depleted in approximately the same amount)
- Hypotonic (sodium loss is > water loss)
- Hypertonic (water loss is > sodium loss)

Isotonic and hypotonic dehydration can also be divided into severity:
- Mild (5%): dry mucous membranes
- Moderate (10%): ill child, sunken eyes and fontanelles, poor peripheral perfusion, oliguria
- Severe (10–15%): shock i.e. tachycardia, hypotension, oliguria/anuria, hyperventilation (respiratory compensation for associated metabolic acidosis) and decreased level of consciousness

Mild cases can be managed at home with 'oral re-hydration solution' (ORS) as long as parents can cope with clear guidelines. Moderate to severe cases need admission to consider intravenous fluid replacement. The signs of hypertonic dehydration may be less obvious.

Management

- Initially 24 hours of ORS for example Dioralyte containing glucose and electrolytes. Ileal absorption of glucose draws sodium and water into the enterocytes. Ideally breast-feeding should continue if tolerated.
- Small volumes of ORS given frequently is more likely to be effective
- Monitor fluid balance: daily weighing, assessing fluid balance frequency of wet nappies etc.
- Associated fever can exacerbate dehydration and regular paracetamol along with other methods of temperature control should be considered
- Admit to hospital with moderate to severe dehydration or if the above has failed
- Remember the possibility of secondary lactose intolerance

4. ***Outline methods that may help to lessen the risk of Sudden Infant Death Syndrome (SIDS).***

- Identify high risk babies and institute a programme of increased surveillance by the health visitor with early referral to a Paediatrician in the case of concern e.g. unexplained weight loss
- Apnoea monitors have not been shown to be of benefit, however, transcutaneous oxygen saturation monitors in high risk babies and siblings of affected infants may help, if only to lessen parental anxiety
- Early immunisation against pertussis may also be of some benefit
- Avoiding contact with infected health care workers and older children at GP surveillance clinics by e.g. providing a separate waiting area for young infants
- Encourage the parents to stop smoking
- Teach parents to recognise signs of illness and manage appropriately
- Instruct parents with 'high risk' babies on methods of basic life support
- Breast-feeding
- Infants should sleep in the supine position
- Avoid hyperthermia (prone position, multiple layers, high tog duvet)

5a.   *Describe methods of testing hearing in neonates.*

Methods

- Ask the parents if they think their baby can hear normally or give a specific questionnaire
- Auditory Response Cradle (ARC). This is a computer-assisted assessment of infant response to sound, eye movements or a change in respiration.
- Auditory Brainstem Responses (ABR). This is a more reliable investigation than ARC and involves recording analysis of EEG signals evoked in response to sound.
- Oto Acoustic Emissions (OAE). Is an auditory echo admitted by a normal cochlea.

NB. District policies vary and screening may be either universal or selective for high risk babies only. However, if hearing loss is suspected it is important not to delay referral until the routine seven month hearing test.

5b.   *List risk factors for deafness in newborns.*

Risk factors

- Prematurity/low birth weight
- Ototoxic drugs e.g. aminoglycosides such as gentamicin
- Family history of deafness (genetically determined sensorineural hearing loss). This may be an isolated defect or part of a syndrome, e.g. Waardenburg syndrome, which is an autosomal dominant condition presenting with deafness and a white forelock.
- Craniofacial anomalies e.g. Treacher-Collins syndrome, cleft palate
- Syndromes with increased association e.g. Down's syndrome
- Birth trauma resulting in severe asphyxia/anoxia and manifesting later as cerebral palsy
- Congenital infection e.g. rubella, CMV and syphilis
- Hyperbilirubinaemia
- Meningitis or encephalitis
- Head injury – secondary to NAI

6.   *Advise a father how to help his children cope with the impending death of their terminally ill mother.*

As the mother has only a few weeks/months to live, it is vital to involve her as much as she is able. If she is still at home, try to keep the routine as normal as possible. If she is in hospital or in a hospice, prepare them before their visit, explain that mum may be 'hooked up to tubes and wires' etc., and that she may not be as attentive as normal or not her usual self. Visits should be frequent but brief to avoid tiring.

Explain the nature and cause of their mother's illness and the possibility of her dying, appropriate to his children's ages. Encourage them to help in her care, just in small ways (not with bed-pans).

With the parents permission inform the school/teacher that they might expect some behavioural problems, so that they are prepared to react sympathetically.

Plan for grief reactions e.g. regression or emotional problems and expect separation anxiety and concern regarding the health of dad and other family members. When the mother has died reassure the children that she is not suffering anymore and that she has gone to a better place e.g. heaven or whatever is appropriate for their cultural beliefs. Encourage them to talk about their mother and keep photographs and momentos around the house. Continually emphasise that they are not responsible for her death.

Attend the funeral and wake and seek support from the GP, Health Visitor, religious 'leader'/priest, extended family and friends, or even formal counselling if required (family therapy, child psychologist). When mourning is over it may be helpful to ask a prominent female (e.g. friend/aunt) to be a 'mother figure', but emphasise that they are not a replacement.

7. **Outline your management of a two-month-old infant with a head circumference on the 97th centile.**

History

- Ante-natal
  Were there any problems?
  Was mum diabetic? (pre-existing or gestational)
  Was the ultrasound scan normal?
  Did the baby have intra-uterine growth retardation?
- Birth – normal vaginal delivery or a Caesarean section and if so why?
- Post natal
  Was the baby well or was he admitted to the Special Care Baby Unit, and if so why?
  Has he been symptomatic/asymptomatic over the last 8 weeks (feeding/behaviour/development)?
  Does mum think he can see/hear?
- Family history
  Any predisposing conditions? e.g. familial megalencephaly
  What are the parents' head circumferences?

Examination

- Plot the height, weight and head circumference since birth – are they all on the 97th centile or do they cross a centile? (corrected for gestation).
- General – dysmorphic, jaundiced, dehydrated, febrile? Is the baby alert and well or not?
- Full examination including neurological – is the baby floppy or hypertonic? Is there asymmetry of his reflexes/movements?
- Look for features of raised intracranial pressure e.g. hydrocephalus/sun-setting eyes, bulging fontanelle, widely separated sutures, irritability, vomiting, papilloedema
- Development: gross motor, fine motor and vision, social development, language and hearing

Differential diagnosis

- A large baby with a proportionally large head
- A normal/small baby with a dis-proportionally large head

In an asymptomatic baby, an innocent explanation is likely, and it is reasonable to simply monitor the child for changes. However, a symptomatic baby, with or without signs of raised ICP needs urgent referral to a Paediatrician for further investigation e.g. cranial USS, CT or MRI scan.

8a. List the common causes of faecal soiling in a 5-year-old boy.

Differential diagnosis

- Delayed maturation of bowel control
- Constipation (chronic) with overflow diarrhoea
- Encopresis: primarily of psychogenic origin
- Faecal incontinence: secondary to neurological problems such as spina bifida
- Pervasive developmental delay
- Gastro-enteritis resulting in profuse diarrhoea

8b. Discuss your management of this problem.

History

- Duration, primary, or if secondary, what is the child's normal bowel habit?
- Is the child otherwise well or has he had a recent infection with vomiting?
- What is the child's diet and what methods have been tried already?
- Drug history, including dose/of laxatives, frequency?
- Past medical history
  Does the child suffer from some form of chronic illness?
  Does the child have any developmental delay or behavioural problems?
- Social history: family stresses, bereavement, marital conflict, illness etc.
- Is there associated enuresis?

Examination

A full examination including abdomen, anus, +/- rectum.

Investigations

Abdominal X-ray, +/- barium enema or +/- referral for rectal biopsy.

Management

- Exclude an organic cause (learning difficulties, constipation, gastro-enteritis etc.)
- Explanation of the problem to the child
- Introduce a record and reward system
- Put a step under the toilet seat to relax the perineum while seated or use a child seat
- Put books/story tapes in the toilet to 'make it fun'
- Introduce training programme i.e. encourage the child to use the toilet approximately 15-20 minutes after a meal (preferably at home)
- If constipated try dietary advice
  Dioctyl (softener), senna (stimulant)
  Picolax (if above fails)
  The child may require a microlax enema and/or glycerine suppositories, however this is rare, or anal dilatation under a general anaesthetic
- Stress to the child that they must take personal responsibility
- Modify the parental response and support the parents as sometimes the child is not actually the patient. Family therapy/counselling may be appropriate.
- Follow-up with support and supervision for one to two years
- More complex family psychosocial issues may be involved and psychiatric referral or inpatient treatment may be necessary if the above measures prove inadequate.

9. *Outline your management of a three-year-old boy whose withdrawn behaviour at play school is causing his teachers concern.*

A full assessment requires good background knowledge. What do staff mean by 'withdrawn'? It is vital with the parents permission, to obtain a report from play school and also a health visitor report, which should include details of previous visits, behaviour of the child in the home environment and any problems concerning the child's siblings. Then arrange a review with the parents and the child together.

History

- Ante-natal/delivery/SCBU i.e. are there any risk factors which impair bonding?
- Do the parents have any concerns over the physical/mental health of the child. Is there any history of features suggestive of autism?
- Is there a history of chronic illness with numerous hospital admissions? Is there developmental delay?
- Is the child on any medication that may affect his behaviour?
- Is there any family history of chronic illness/psychiatric illness or behavioural problems?
- Social history
  Family dynamics, marital conflicts?
  Any stressors e.g. financial, eviction, illness, bereavement
  History of parental use of drugs, alcohol abuse, psychiatric disorder
  Are there any other risk factors for clinical abuse?
  Consider the possibility that the parents were themselves abused as children.

Examination

- Note the child's general appearance i.e. 'frozen watchfulness', thin, bruising, febrile?
- A full examination 'looking for signs of' organic disease
- A developmental examination,
- Chart his head circumference, height and weight. Is he thriving?
- Examine for signs of autism

Investigations

- Hearing test
- Visual assessment
- Refer to the community paediatrician for a multi-disciplinary assessment +/- a case conference if appropriate
- Check with the social services department to see if he is on the child protection register

10a. **Outline your management of a two-week-old boy whose Guthrie tests have shown a TSH > 100 mu/L.**

A raised TSH suggests hypothyroidism. It is important to contact the parents and arrange a consultation with them as soon as possible, ideally that day. First ensure the baby is well i.e. ABC etc. Take a history of the pregnancy, the birth and enquire about symptoms of hypothyroidism in the baby e.g. lethargy, prolonged jaundice, hypotonia, poor feeding, noisy breathing, constipation, hoarse cry, hypothermia and bradycardia. Has there been any maternal ingestion of goitrogens during the pregnancy? e.g. iodine-containing cough mixture, anti-thyroid drugs.

The child needs urgent referral to hospital for further investigations including formal TSH and T4, serum T3 and thyroid antibodies. More specialised tests may **rarely** be required later on e.g. radioisotope scanning with technetium or radioactive iodine which detects the presence of thyroid tissue, including 'ectopic' tissue. Bone age should also be assessed – X-ray of the distal femoral epiphysis in term infants will usually demonstrate calcified ossification centres, however this will not be apparent in infants with congenital hypothyroidism.

If treatment is not started by three months irreversible brain damage ensues with other clinical features of hypothyroidism e.g. coarse facies, goitre (although this is unusual as most are athyroid), delayed bone age, retarded development and growth failure. Therefore thyroxine should be started as soon as possible initially at a dose of 10 mcg/kg daily and adjusted accordingly to keep the serum thyroxine at the upper range of normal for age (TSH levels take some months to fall).

10b.   Discuss your initial counselling of the parents.

- Discuss the reason for performing routine Guthrie tests and explain the significance of this result
- Discuss the possible causes and how this may affect the child with or without treatment
- Discuss how this will affect the rest of the family and the potential risk to future children (very rare, usually sporadic thyroid agenesis)
- Emphasise the need for urgent referral and discuss the possible investigations and treatments
- Outline the prognosis and importance of compliance with treatment
- Provide contact numbers for various self-help groups
- Liaise with the consultant paediatrician regarding further hospital outpatient follow-up once discharged

CASE COMMENTARY 1

1. As their GP how would you respond to this information?

It is important that the GP reviews the child as soon as possible. Initially assess any concerns the parents may have and frankly discuss the issues raised by the Health Visitor. A full history is necessary, including an antenatal history, looking for risk factors e.g. IUGR, any problems with the birth and of course a developmental history. Does mum think that Simon can see and hear etc.? A full examination is also necessary to look for features of Down's syndrome (flat facial profile, protruding tongue etc) and particularly to exclude any potential life threatening congenital heart disease (cyanosis/heart murmur) and that, despite his feeding problems, he is not dehydrated or malnourished.

Early diagnosis and intervention are essential to maximise the child's potential, therefore if a handicap is suspected by anyone, immediate referral to a paediatrician should be arranged for definitive diagnosis.

The Consultant Community Paediatrician is generally the best to organise assessment as he can arrange karyotyping or a referral to a Geneticist if there is still doubt, but also has access to the full multi-disciplinary team for optimal follow-up. It is vital to keep the parents informed at all stages and arrange to see them again after Simon's assessment to review the findings.

2. How would you counsel the parents at this time?

Both parents should be told the diagnosis together, and the likely development of their child discussed. 'Guilt' is a common reaction and it is important to emphasise that it is not their fault. Find out what information has been given to them by the hospital and go through it with them, answering any questions or worries they may have. Introduction to the Down's Children Association and information about developmental programmes to stimulate early progress may help parents to adopt a positive approach. Provide practical help and support. Also discuss genetic counselling when appropriate and the risk of recurrence.

3. How might you help them at this point?

Although the parents initially accept the situation, prolonged counselling and support for the family is often required as the parents come to terms with Simon's handicap. It is important to ascertain exactly why they feel a 'home' would be the best solution and if mum really agrees or has been pressurised into it. It is important to advise them against making any major decisions while they have still barely come to terms with the situation.

Sympathetic listening is vital; many parents will express anger (at professionals/God) as part of the grief reaction for the loss of their 'normal' child. Lack of information is the most frequent complaint, so they may be helped by contact with self help groups who offer support from other parents (an approachable mum can frequently help them accept their own often very loveable Down's child). These groups also provide additional information about aids, respite care and new therapies. Discuss the various possibilities for respite care e.g. to a purpose run unit, to family/friends, organised holidays and residential placement. If the main concern is financial, reassure and advise about allowances, local charitable funds etc. Refer for genetic counselling if appropriate.

Optimise learning opportunities from an early age, development stimulation programmes such as 'Portage', which involves parents working with therapists in helping developmentally-delayed children to acquire skills and the parents to learn ways of managing future potential behavioural problems. At a later date help parents plan for the future by discussing leaving school and subsequent care. Provide information about adult training centres, sheltered employment, day centres etc.

CASE COMMENTARY 2

1. What are the possible explanations behind Karl's change of behaviour and how would you initially manage this problem?

Karl's likely differential diagnoses include drug or alcohol abuse, a secondary reaction to acute life events or stress, psychiatric illness, a behavioural disorder or simply getting in with the 'wrong crowd'.

Initial management should include involving the school, with the parents permission, particularly the school nurse or counsellor. Family therapy may also be of benefit, or if necessary referral to a child psychiatrist. Other help may be achieved via the social worker or from various support agencies.

2. What would you discuss with the family at this point?

To investigate Karl a detailed history should be obtained from the parents and Karl e.g. what was he like before? What has happened over the last five months? (life events/bereavements/moves) and why now? What are the family's child rearing practises and have his siblings had similar problems? Is it a large chaotic family and are there any parental problems? (psychiatric illness/discords/criminality). Are there significant socio-cultural influences (peer groups/poor housing/low income/poor school)? Are they an isolated family with no close knit community around them?

Obtaining a school report (with parental permission) would also be helpful in assessing Karl. Also ask about any significant past medical history (e.g. multiple separations due to frequent hospital admissions), developmental history and especially a drug history. You should perform a full examination including a neurological and mental state examination. Simple blood tests may be of use including a full blood count, liver function test, and if seen acutely, levels for Toluene, Acetone and other drugs should be considered.

3. What are the perils to which Karl is being exposed?

Karl is in danger of falling into a criminal lifestyle. He is at risk from peer pressure, further experimentation leading to addiction and morbidity from general health deterioration, hallucinations, delusions, hepatic and renal damage. There are also potential fatal consequences to Karl's actions. Drug overdose may lead to CNS depression and convulsions; accidents or other trauma; aspiration leading to respiratory depression, anoxia, vagal inhibition and finally arrhythmias and ultimately death.

4. What is your specific management of this problem and what other professional help may be required?

Ninety five per cent of children experimenting with solvents only do it a few times and it can be dealt with by the GP or local Child Guidance clinic with help from other professionals e.g. social worker. As the GP you should arrange to see Karl alone at first and discuss confidentially with him the facts as you see it and ask for his response. Involve the parents to arrange a plan of action that may include a weekly assessment, for a month initially and then less frequently as he progresses. Limit Karl's pocket money, chaperone him to and from school and remove alcohol and solvents from the house. Prevent him from mixing with a bad crowd, changing school if necessary. Get consent to deal with the school year heads and consider referring him to an activity based self-help group. A Probation Officer may be involved if any criminality has occurred.

If there is no improvement with the above regime, Karl may need referral to the Child Guidance Clinic, various voluntary organisations, child and family psychiatric teams for family therapy, or even a Drug Dependency Unit. The school and the police may help improve education in public health by organising talks at the school and the government may enforce restrictions on the sale of solvents to children under 18 years of age.

5. What are the prospects for Karl and his family?

If Karl has not developed an addiction to solvents then with adequate intervention, a united front from the parents and a lot of support, prognosis may be good. However, with a five-month history of increasingly bad behaviour and drug abuse, probable addiction (turning to crime to finance his addiction) then his prognosis is poor. Further experimentation is likely resulting in significant morbidity and mortality.

60 questions: time allowed 2 hours
Indicate your correct answers with a tick in the boxes provided

2.1 Acute renal failure (ARF)

❏ A gentamicin is a cause of prerenal failure
❏ B may be caused by haemolytic uraemic syndrome
❏ C may be complicated by convulsions or tetany
❏ D management should include a high protein diet
❏ E an indication for dialysis is a plasma urea > 54 mmol/l

2.2 False-negative tuberculin tests can result

❏ A with concurrent infectious mononucleosis
❏ B with concurrent upper respiratory tract viral infection
❏ C if given within one month of immunisation with the MMR vaccine
❏ D with concurrent sarcoidosis
❏ E if given within one month of immunisation with the pertussis vaccine

2.3 Which of these definitions is correct?

❏ A the 'incidence' of influenza is much lower than its 'prevalence'
❏ B the 'perinatal mortality' is the number of stillbirths and deaths within the first week of life per 1000 total births
❏ C 'stillbirth rate' is the number of stillbirths per 1000 total births
❏ D 'neonatal mortality rate' (NMR) is the number of deaths up to one month of age per 1000 total births
❏ E 'infant mortality rate' (IMR) is the number of deaths under one year of age per 1000 total births

2.4 Regarding screening criteria

❏ A a screening test should have low sensitivity and specificity
❏ B acceptable screening tests should give a yield of at least 1 in 100,000
❏ C screening tests should be inexpensive
❏ D effective screening tests are available for the majority of conditions
❏ E screening must be a continuous process

2.5   With regard to paediatric resuscitation

❑ A   most cardiac arrests in children are due to respiratory arrest
❑ B   a Breslow tape is of no use
❑ C   cardiac arrest secondary to drowning has a particularly poor prognosis
❑ D   intraosseous access is suitable for children up to six years of age
❑ E   a cuffed endotracheal tube should always be used to prevent regurgitation and aspiration

2.6   Maternal risk factors for an increased perinatal mortality and morbidity include

❑ A   age between 16–35 years
❑ B   short stature
❑ C   a birth interval of 18–36 months
❑ D   a twin pregnancy
❑ E   a previous ectopic pregnancy

2.7   Apgar scores

❑ A   a heart rate of < 100 scores 1
❑ B   approximately 45% of all babies whose Apgar score is < 4 at 5 minutes will die
❑ C   are recorded at 0, 1 and 5 minutes
❑ D   are not used in intubated babies
❑ E   a blue baby scores 0

2.8   Features linked to depression in a child of ten years may include

❑ A   diabetes mellitus
❑ B   epilepsy
❑ C   primary enuresis
❑ D   abdominal pain
❑ E   recent vandalism

2.9 Plagiocephaly

☐ A is often associated with babies who are consistently put into the cot on the same side

☐ B may present with torticollis at six months to three years

☐ C is associated with craniosynostosis

☐ D has an increased incidence of epilepsy

☐ E generally spontaneously improves with time

2.10 Features of a headache that would alert you to the diagnoses of serious intracranial pathology are

☐ A transient ataxia, hemiparesis or aphasia

☐ B recent onset of a squint

☐ C if it wakens the child at night and is most severe first thing in the morning

☐ D relief from implementing an 'exclusion diet' (i.e. chocolate, cheese, milk etc.)

☐ E deterioration in school performance

2.11 Regarding congenital heart disease

☐ A patent ductus arteriosus (PDA) is more common in premature infants than in term infants

☐ B children with coarctation of the aorta typically squat after exercise

☐ C cyanosis is more obvious in the anaemic child

☐ D atrial septal defect (ASD) has a soft ejection systolic murmur with a wide fixed split of the second heart sound

☐ E clubbing develops at around one year of age in children with cyanotic cardiac lesions

2.12 Neurofibromatosis type 1 (NF1)

☐ A is an autosomal recessive disorder

☐ B presents in childhood

☐ C often presents with bilateral acoustic neuroma

☐ D may develop optic nerve glioma

☐ E may develop kyphoscoliosis

2.13   Congenital dislocation of the hip

❏   A   is more common in boys
❏   B   occurs in 5–20 per 1000 live births
❏   C   affects the right hip more than the left
❏   D   the diagnosis should be confirmed by USS
❏   E   is associated with a breech presentation

2.14   Tuberous sclerosis

❏   A   is an autosomal dominant condition
❏   B   is associated with infantile spasms
❏   C   often presents with adenoma sebaceum in infancy
❏   D   Wood's lamp examination is unnecessary in this condition
❏   E   affected children may have a characteristic 'white streak' in their hair

2.15   Acute epiglottitis

❏   A   is caused by a parainfluenza virus
❏   B   should be diagnosed by checking for the typical cherry red swelling of the epiglottis
❏   C   is associated with drooling
❏   D   has a characteristic barking cough
❏   E   should have an elective endotracheal intubation

2.16   Wilms' nephroblastoma

❏   A   at presentation over 80% of children have metastases
❏   B   may be familial
❏   C   is resistant to radiotherapy
❏   D   can present with failure to thrive ± hemihypertrophy
❏   E   may be associated with GU malformations

2.17   Known side-effects of carbamazepine include

❏   A   aplastic anaemia
❏   B   rickets
❏   C   ataxia
❏   D   transient hair loss
❏   E   rash

2.18   A normal 18-month-old child

❏   A   can build a tower of eight bricks
❏   B   should be able to copy a vertical line
❏   C   will hold a pen in a 'tripod' grip
❏   D   enjoys looking at books, and will help turn the pages two or
            three at a time
❏   E   can copy a circle

2.19   Features of cystic fibrosis include

❏   A   rectal prolapse
❏   B   prolonged neonatal jaundice
❏   C   digital clubbing
❏   D   failure to thrive
❏   E   Pseudomonas chest infection

2.20   Known side-effects of clonazepam

❏   A   salivary and bronchial hypersecretion
❏   B   nystagmus
❏   C   somnolence and hypotonia
❏   D   reversible leukopenia
❏   E   acne

2.21   Roseola infantum

❏   A   presents with a rash on the first day
❏   B   has an incubation period of approximately 5–15 days
❏   C   is commonly due to herpes virus type 6
❏   D   is also known as '5th disease'
❏   E   is associated with pneumonia

2.22   Causes of short stature include

❏   A   Noonan syndrome
❏   B   Soto's syndrome
❏   C   Turner's syndrome
❏   D   Klinefelter's syndrome
❏   E   Marfan's syndrome

2.23   Causes of tall stature include

❑   A   constitutional
❑   B   homocysteinuria
❑   C   hyperthyroidism
❑   D   pseudohypoparathyroidism
❑   E   Cushing's syndrome

2.24   The floppy infant syndrome may be caused by

❑   A   an acute infection in a normal infant
❑   B   Down's syndrome
❑   C   Prader–Willi syndrome
❑   D   cerebral palsy
❑   E   Werdnig–Hoffmann disease

2.25   Cystic fibrosis

❑   A   affects approximately 1 in 2000 live births in the UK
❑   B   has an X-linked inheritance
❑   C   may present with meconium ileus
❑   D   is associated with delayed puberty
❑   E   is associated with nasal polyposis

2.26   With regard to immunisations

❑   A   live attenuated vaccines include measles, mumps, rubella and
          BCG
❑   B   the vaccines comprising inactivated organisms include
          pertussis and 'Sabin' (poliomyelitis – OPV)
❑   C   Hib is known as a 'component vaccine' and provokes a cell-
          mediated response
❑   D   vaccinations to tetanus and diphtheria comprise inactivated
          toxins
❑   E   vaccines comprising inactivated organisms and toxins
          stimulate an antibody or antitoxin IgM primary response

2.27   Common features of cystic fibrosis include

❏   A   anorexia
❏   B   steatorrhoea
❏   C   a positive sweat test, where the concentration of sweat sodium is > 70 mmol/l
❏   D   an increased incidence in the Chinese
❏   E   male impotence

2.28   Treatment of asthma

❏   A   aminophylline cannot be given if the child is already on regular oral theophylline
❏   B   cromoglycate is a useful agent in the treatment of acute asthma
❏   C   inhalers deliver less than 5% of the drug to the lungs
❏   D   the incidence of oral candidiasis can be reduced if steroids are inhaled via a spacer device
❏   E   regular inhaled low dose steroids do not result in growth retardation

2.29   Conditions that may result in a false-positive sweat test include

❏   A   Addison's disease
❏   B   hypothyroidism
❏   C   diabetes mellitus
❏   D   nephrogenic diabetes insipidus
❏   E   bronchiectasis

2.30   A normal 3-year-old child

❏   A   can build a tower of eight bricks
❏   B   can imitate a three brick bridge
❏   C   can copy a square
❏   D   will hold a pen with a mature grip
❏   E   cannot copy a circle

2.31   The 1993 Education Act

❏   A   defines a child with special educational needs (SEN) as one who has a learning difficulty that requires special educational provision to be made

❏   B   children whose language of the home is different from the one in which they will be taught may be considered to have a learning difficulty

❏   C   children with SEN should be taught in special schools

❏   D   a statement of SEN should be made and reviewed regularly

❏   E   special educational provision includes any educational provision given to a child under two years of age

2.32   Concerning accidents

❏   A   they are the single largest cause of death in children between 1 and 14 years

❏   B   60% of all childhood deaths are due to accidents

❏   C   the commonest fatal accidents are due to falls

❏   D   approximately 15% of all children per year attend A&E because of an accidental injury

❏   E   boys and girls have an equal incidence

2.33   Causes of neonatal unconjugated hyperbilirubinaemia include

❏   A   rhesus incompatibility

❏   B   extrahepatic biliary atresia

❏   C   hypothyroidism

❏   D   glucose-6-phosphate dehydrogenase deficiency

❏   E   choledochal cysts

2.34   Examples of primary prevention include

❏   A   cycling helmets

❏   B   stair gates

❏   C   teaching children road safety from a young age

❏   D   smoke alarms

❏   E   child proof catches on cupboards

2.35   Examples of secondary prevention include

❏   A   seat belts
❏   B   blister packs for prescription drugs
❏   C   teaching parents first aid skills
❏   D   fire extinguishers kept in the house
❏   E   speed limits

2.36   Bilirubin toxicity

❏   A   is caused by free unconjugated bilirubin which is lipid soluble and therefore readily diffuses across brain cell membranes
❏   B   kernicterus only occurs when the serum bilirubin exceeds 380 mmol/l
❏   C   symptoms include hypotonia and lethargy
❏   D   if the baby survives, long-term sequelae include choreoathetoid cerebral palsy and high frequency nerve deafness
❏   E   phototherapy uses a narrow spectrum blue light of wavelength 450–475 nm

2.37   The Dubowitz system for assessment of gestational age include the following external criteria:

❏   A   nipple formation
❏   B   ear firmness
❏   C   nail development
❏   D   presence of eyelashes
❏   E   breast size

2.38   Congenital rubella syndrome includes

❏   A   deafness
❏   B   microphthalmia
❏   C   cardiac defects
❏   D   cerebral palsy
❏   E   saddle nose

2.39 **Infants born to poorly controlled diabetic mothers may have**

- ❏ A Erb's palsy
- ❏ B sacral agenesis
- ❏ C hypomagnesaemia
- ❏ D hypercalcaemia
- ❏ E anaemia

2.40 **The following drugs are safe in breast-feeding:**

- ❏ A thyroxine
- ❏ B digoxin
- ❏ C nitrazepam
- ❏ D cimetidine
- ❏ E chlorpheniramine

2.41 **Common causes of epistaxis in children include**

- ❏ A nose picking
- ❏ B hypertension
- ❏ C upper respiratory tract infection
- ❏ D atrophic rhinitis
- ❏ E foreign bodies

2.42 **With regard to adoption**

- ❏ A the adopted child takes on the nationality of his adoptive parents
- ❏ B applicants must be aged 18 or over
- ❏ C the natural parents must give their informed consent before the adoption can proceed
- ❏ D the child must live with the adoptive parents for six months before the order is finalised
- ❏ E at age 16 an adopted child is entitled to his original birth certificate

2.43   Foster care

❑   A   short-term fostering is usually less than 18 months
❑   B   long-term fostering is preferred for younger children
❑   C   is more likely to be successful if there are children of a similar age in the placement family
❑   D   there is usually a limit of three foster children per family
❑   E   children in long-term foster care require a six monthly medical examination

2.44   Concerning dentition

❑   A   there are 32 deciduous teeth
❑   B   teething causes fever, irritability and excessive salivation
❑   C   children do not have the hand-eye co-ordination to adequately clean their teeth until approximately 8–10 years of age
❑   D   the first tooth to appear is generally a lower central incisor
❑   E   malocclusion may result from thumb sucking

2.45   In the treatment of asthma

❑   A   oral salbutamol syrup is useful in the treatment of infants and toddlers
❑   B   a plastic coffee cup may be used as a spacer device
❑   C   inhaled drugs cannot be effectively delivered to children under two years of age
❑   D   a three year old can use dry powder inhalers
❑   E   a spacer device is unsuitable in children over ten years

2.46   Urinary tract infection (UTI)

❑   A   may present with vomiting, irritability and feeding problems
❑   B   should be investigated during or after their second UTI
❑   C   urine specimens can be stored at 0–4°C for up to 24 hours
❑   D   the presence of pyuria proves a UTI
❑   E   obesity predisposes to UTIs in girls

2.47   Risk factors for sudden infant death syndrome (SIDS) include

❑   A   female sex
❑   B   twins
❑   C   bottle feeding
❑   D   previous history of a sibling dying from SIDS
❑   E   supine sleeping position

2.48   Management of urinary tract infections

❑   A   amoxycillin is the first-line treatment in children
❑   B   prophylactic antibiotics are given four times daily for one month
❑   C   includes avoiding constipation
❑   D   asymptomatic bacteriuria should always be treated with appropriate antibiotics
❑   E   may involve surgery

2.49   Causes of haematuria include

❑   A   exercise
❑   B   idiopathic
❑   C   allergy
❑   D   meatal stenosis
❑   E   malaria

2.50   Vesico-ureteric reflux (VUR)

❑   A   should be routinely screened for in all children under five years
❑   B   10% of children with VUR will develop renal scarring
❑   C   grade II VUR involves urine refluxing into the kidney on micturition only
❑   D   if severe may require an endoscopic submucosal Teflon injection
❑   E   requires monitoring with serial USS

2.51   Scabies

❏   A   is caused by the *Sarcoptes scabiei* mite
❏   B   burrows usually involve the interdigital webs or flexor aspects of the wrists, while sparing the face and scalps of infants
❏   C   symptomatic family members only need to be treated
❏   D   itching is usually worse at night
❏   E   persistent pruritus two weeks later implies failure of treatment

2.52   Obesity

❏   A   is associated with growth hormone deficiency
❏   B   may be complicated by Blount's disease
❏   C   is associated with Lawrence–Moon–Biedl syndrome
❏   D   all obese healthy children are tall for their age
❏   E   is associated with hyperparathyroidism

2.53   Cerebral palsy

❏   A   is a progressive condition
❏   B   has a prevalence of 2.5 in 1000
❏   C   is associated with a mental handicap in 70–80% of cases
❏   D   is due to perinatal hypoxic-ischaemic injury in the majority of cases
❏   E   may present with clumsiness

2.54   Management of epilepsy includes

❏   A   ketogenic diet
❏   B   discouraging swimming
❏   C   protective helmets should be worn while cycling alone on open roads
❏   D   surgery
❏   E   education in normal schools

2.55   Regarding spastic hemiplegia

❏   A   the legs are more severely affected than the arms
❏   B   it may result from an infarct of the cortex or internal capsule
❏   C   almost all affected children walk by school age
❏   D   one leg may be shorter than the other
❏   E   it characteristically results in learning difficulties

2.56 **Causes of childhood seizures include**

- ❏ A tuberous sclerosis
- ❏ B porphyria
- ❏ C lead poisoning
- ❏ D hypoglycaemia
- ❏ E neurofibromatosis

2.57 **Causes of constipation include**

- ❏ A congenital absence of intestinal autonomic ganglion cells of the Auerbach and Messier plexus
- ❏ B dehydration
- ❏ C hypocalcaemia
- ❏ D hypothyroidism
- ❏ E over-enthusiastic potty training

2.58 **Phenylketonuria**

- ❏ A is an autosomal dominant condition
- ❏ B is associated with infantile spasms
- ❏ C is detected using the Guthrie test at approximately day six
- ❏ D will result in mental retardation if the diagnosis is delayed
- ❏ E normal infants may be damaged *in utero* if their affected mothers do not maintain their dietary restrictions throughout the pregnancy

2.59 **With regard to HIV infection**

- ❏ A the risk of vertical transmission in Europe is approximately 50%
- ❏ B breast-feeding should be avoided in developed countries
- ❏ C it is a notifiable disease
- ❏ D Pneumovax is contraindicated
- ❏ E testing for HIV antibodies helps to exclude neonatal congenital infection

2.60 **The following are notifiable diseases:**

- ❏ A AIDS
- ❏ B mumps
- ❏ C tuberculosis
- ❏ D rubella
- ❏ E malaria

SHORT NOTE QUESTIONS – PAPER 2

10 questions: time allowed 1 hour 30 minutes
Write short notes of the following subjects. Conciseness will be
beneficial. Lists are acceptable.

1. Advise the parents of a 10-year-old boy with normally well controlled insulin dependent diabetes who develops a febrile illness.

2. What are the characteristics of a child with a febrile convulsion that would suggest an increased risk of developing epilepsy?

3. How would you prevent the spread of head lice? Discuss methods of eradication.

4. A seven-week-old baby has become inconsolable every evening for the last twelve days. What are the possible diagnoses and how would you manage this case?

5. What are the problems encountered with distraction hearing tests?

6. How would you assess a five-year-old boy whose mother feels he is excessively 'clumsy' and has poor writing skills? Outline the general management plan.

7. What are the symptoms and signs of a complex partial seizure (temporal lobe) in a school age child? Make a list of possible differential diagnoses.

8a. List valid indications for performing a circumcision.
8b The majority of circumcisions (excluding religious/cultural reasons) are not performed for preputial disease. Why is this the case?

9. Write short notes on the Emergency Protection Order and obtaining consent for children under 16 years.

10. What is the differential diagnosis of persistent jaundice of a one-month-old infant? List useful investigations.

CASE COMMENTARIES – PAPER 2

Two questions: time allowed 1 hour 30 minutes
Read the following case history carefully. Then answer all the
questions below. Please start your answer on a separate page.

CASE COMMENTARY 1

Emma, an 18-month-girl, is brought to the Accident and Emergency Department by her parents. They had found her fitting and are now unable to rouse her. Their GP had started amoxycillin the day before for otitis media associated with fever. She was previously fit and well with no history of convulsions. On examination she is unconscious reacting only to painful stimuli. Her temperature is 36.5 °C, she has a regular pulse of 70/min and her respiratory rate is 18/min.

1.   **What is your initial management of Emma?**

2.   **Give your differential diagnosis. What are the most appropriate investigations you would order?**

A more detailed history is taken which reveals that Emma's dad has recently been diagnosed as an insulin dependent diabetic. Emma's mum is a trained nurse, however her husband's work has just moved them to the area and she has not yet found steady employment. Emma is their first child. She is found to have a blood glucose of 1.7 mmol/L and recovers quickly following intravenous glucose and hydrocortisone. She is admitted and over the next ten days has three more convulsions all associated with hypoglycaemia.

3.   **What is the probable diagnosis?**

4.   **What is the most important investigation now?**

A case conference is organised.

5.   **Outline the points to be made at the case conference and the possible ways this family can be helped.**

CASE COMMENTARY 2

Sarah is the 18-month-old daughter of a 30-year-old factory worker and his 26-year-old wife. During an appointment with the health visitor mother mentions that Sarah is not sleeping well at night, which is causing considerable stress for the whole family. They have tried leaving her in her own cot but she cries constantly until the parents either have to pick her up and put her into bed with them or stay with her for long periods of time until she settles. Dad works early shifts and feels his chronic tiredness is making him perform badly at work. Sarah shares a room with her 5-year-old sister who has recently started having tantrums in the morning insisting she is too tired to go to school. They live in a two-bedroom council flat. Sarah's grandparents are nearby and very supportive. Mother eventually confides that she may be pregnant again and is unsure what to do.

1.   What history, examination and investigations would be most appropriate at this stage to help diagnose and manage this problem?

2.   What problems might Sarah's parents have and how will they affect the situation?

3.   What advice would you give the parents handling this sleep problem? What other help is available (night sedation is shown to be of no benefit)?

MULTIPLE CHOICE QUESTION PAPER 2 – ANSWERS

2.1 **Answers: B C E**

Acute renal failure occurs with sudden disturbance of renal function resulting in a decreased urine output with a rising serum urea and creatinine. There are three main causes.

1. Prerenal: due to hypovolaemia (e.g. burns) or hypotension (e.g. septicaemia)
2. Renal: (e.g. haemolytic uraemic syndrome, acute glomerulonephritis and nephrotoxins (i.e. gentamicin)).
3. Post renal: due to congenital (e.g. urethral valves) or acquired (e.g. renal calculi) obstructive uropathy

Management involves resuscitation, fluid restriction, correction of electrolytes, i.v. antibiotics if septic, a high calorie/low protein diet (TPN may be necessary) and possibly dialysis. Indications for dialysis include a diuretic resistant hypervolaemia with hypertension and pulmonary oedema, a plasma urea > 54 mmol/l, hyperkalaemia, metabolic acidosis or a dialysable nephrotoxin. ARF may be complicated by convulsions and tetany, which are secondary to the associated hypocalcaemia and hypomagnesaemia.

2.2 **Answers: A B C D**

False-negative tuberculin tests can result if given within one month of immunisation with MMR because it is a live vaccine and provokes a cell-mediated response that may therefore result in a suboptimal reaction to skin testing. False-negatives also occur with sarcoidosis, Hodgkin's lymphoma, HIV infection and other immunosuppressant diseases or therapies. The pertussis vaccine is inactive and therefore does not affect skin testing.

2.3 **Answers: B C**

The 'incidence' is the number of new cases occurring during a specified period in a defined population, whereas the 'prevalence' is the number of cases at any particular time or during a specified period of time in a defined population. Therefore an acute illness will have a high incidence, but low prevalence, whereas the annual incidence of a chronic illness will be much lower than its prevalence. Both are expressed as a rate per 1000 of the population.

The NMR is the number of deaths of live born babies up to one month of age per 1000 live births and the IMR is the number of deaths of all children under one year of age per 1000 live births.

2.4   **Answers: C E**

Screening tests should have a high sensitivity (i.e. few false negatives) and high specificity (i.e. few false positives). Screening tests should be inexpensive, however calculation of the true cost should include the money saved by detection of the disease at an early stage. Therefore 'cost-effective' is probably a more accurate term. The screening test should also be easy to perform, acceptable to the patient, repeatable and producing a yield of at least 1 in 10,000 positive diagnoses of a treatable condition. Effective screening tests are available for a limited number of conditions. Ideally the defined condition screened for should be an important one with a recognisable latent or early symptomatic stage and a well-known natural history if untreated. Screening must be a continuous process to be effective and not a 'one-off'. General Practitioners are ideally suited to implement screening tests.

2.5   **Answers: A D**

Cardiac arrest in children has an extremely poor prognosis in the majority of cases and is most frequently due to severe illness or injury resulting in hypoxia, acidosis and respiratory arrest. The few survivors often have neurological sequelae. However, cold water drowning is the one area where prolonged resuscitation after cardiac arrest has had some success.

Finding the correct size of equipment during paediatric resuscitation can be confusing and the Breslow tape is extremely useful at removing the guesswork. From the height, it estimates the child's weight and each 'weight' has a list of appropriate drug dosages, fluid boluses and equipment sizes for easy reference. Cuffed endotracheal tubes should never be used in children, as unlike adults the narrowest diameter is at the level of the cricoid ring, which is susceptible to the pressure effects of the cuff. Intraosseous access is suitable in children up to six years of age and is more recently being accepted as a last resort in older children and adults (sternal i.o. placement).

2.6   **Answers: B D E**

An adverse obstetric history is a risk factor including previous ectopic pregnancy, abortion, antepartum haemorrhage, preterm labour, Caesarean section, perinatal death or congenital abnormality. A birth interval of 18–36 months is associated with the lowest perinatal mortality rare, whereas an interval less than 12 months has the highest. A multiple pregnancy and maternal age greater than 35 years are also risk factors.

2.7   **Answers: A B D**

Score	Pulse	Resp. rate	Muscle tone	Colour	Reflex on suction
0	0	Nil	Limp	White	Nil
1	<100	Slow/ irregular	Limb flexion	Blue	Grimace
2	>100	Regular	Active	Pink	Cough

Apgar scores are usually recorded at 1 minute, 5 minutes and at 5 minute intervals after births.

2.8   **Answers: A B D E**

Depression may often initially present with various psychosomatic symptoms (e.g. abdominal pain, headache). However, the presence of an actual chronic physical disease (e.g. asthma, diabetes) is a predisposing factor and various medications, including steroids and some anticonvulsants can also result in depression. Depression may also present with behavioural problems such as vandalism or drug abuse and younger children may regress, resulting in, for example, secondary enuresis.

2.9   **Answers: A C E**

Plagiocephaly is associated with craniosynostosis and also with babies who have suffered damage to their sternomastoid muscle and consequently develop a sternomastoid tumour (which may present with torticollis). This pulls the head persistently to the affected side resulting in retarded facial growth on that side and hence facial asymmetry. Advice on alternating the head position in the cot generally results in spontaneous improvement over time. If it is secondary to sternomastoid tumour it may also resolve, but may need physiotherapy if it persists. Later treatment involves division of the muscle at the distal end.

2.10   **Answers: B C E**

Migraines are generally preceded by an 'aura' that varies depending on which artery is affected. Vasoconstriction of the cranial artery may result in a transient oculomotor nerve palsy, ataxia, hemiparesis or aphasia. Intracranial pathology usually results in some permanent residual neurology. Migraine sufferers have a positive family history in 80% of cases, whereas acute severe headaches with no past medical or family history are more indicative of intracranial pathology. A significant space-occupying lesion may present with personality change, headaches that wake the child at night and are worse in the morning. Headaches may occur daily, escalating in a crescendo pattern; they may be accompanied by vomiting and a stiff neck and are exacerbated by coughing and bending over. 'Exclusion diets' are of no benefit and are generally part of the management of migrainous headaches, which should also respond to other simple measures such as lying in a darkened room, analgesics and antiemetics.

2.11   **Answers: A D E**

The ductus normally functionally closes within approximately 12 hours of birth and is obliterated over the next 2–3 weeks. Delayed closure is often seen in premature infants, who may require an indomethacin infusion (i.e. a prostaglandin synthetase inhibitor) to hasten the process. Symptomatic PDAs (e.g. failure to thrive, cardiomegaly) require definitive surgery in infancy, whereas the majority are asymptomatic and surgical closure can be deferred until 1–3 years of age.

Squatting after exercise is a classic presentation of Fallot's tetralogy, as the affected children attempt to increase the systemic vascular resistance and thus reduce the right to left shunt. Cyanosis is more difficult to detect clinically in the anaemic child and cyanotic cardiac lesions tend to result in clubbing after about one year of age.

2.12   **Answers: B D E**

Both NF1 and NF2 are autosomal dominant conditions. NF1 presents in childhood, whereas NF2 presents in early adulthood. Bilateral acoustic neuroma is more typical of NF2.

2.13 **Answers: B D E**

One per cent of hips at birth are found to be unstable and are more common on the left (60%) with one in five being bilateral. Risk factors include female sex (80%), family history, breech delivery, first child and history of oligohydramnios.

Screening involves the Ortolani–Barlow manoeuvre with USS of suspicious joints, which shows the shape of the cartilaginous socket and position of the femoral head (X-rays are unhelpful before six weeks). If these tests are positive, neonates should be splinted in abduction for 6–12 weeks with clinical and radiological follow-up at three, six and twelve months. Most hips will have stabilised with conservative methods however, persistent instability will need surgery. This is more likely if initial treatment was delayed.

2.14 **Answers: A B**

Tuberous sclerosis is an autosomal dominant condition with variable penetrance and 80% occurring as new mutations. It is associated with infantile spasms and epilepsy in later childhood. Skin abnormalities include ash-leaf macules, a 'shagreen' patch, periungual fibromata, facial telangiectasia and adenoma sebaceum (facial angiofibroma) which usually develops after puberty. Wood's lamp examination of the child (and parents) clearly shows up areas of ash-leaf depigmentation – the presenting feature in 95% of children. The characteristic 'white streak' of hair is typical of Wardenburg's syndrome.

2.15 **Answers: C E**

Acute epiglottitis is caused by *Haemophilus influenzae* type B. It generally occurs between two to six years of age and the diagnosis is made from the history and classic clinical appearance. Within a few hours of developing a sore throat the child becomes hot, toxic, drooling due to difficulty swallowing, is unable to speak and is petrified. The child is dyspnoeic, has inspiratory stridor, subcostal recession and typically holds his head in hyperextension to keep the airway clear and there is usually no cough. Anything that may increase the child's distress should be avoided as this may precipitate a respiratory arrest requiring an emergency attempt at endotracheal intubation by junior staff. This includes unnecessary investigations, such as a lateral neck X-ray and examination of the throat is absolutely contraindicated. If the condition is suspected an experienced anaesthetist should called to perform an elective endotracheal intubation in a controlled environment, such as theatre.

Croup, in comparison, presents with a longer history, a characteristic barking cough and moderate pyrexia; stridor is harsh and there is no drooling.

2.16   **Answers: B D E**

Wilms' nephroblastoma is the commonest of all childhood malignant tumours accounting for 10% of cases. It presents before five years of age in 80% of children with a median age of 3.5 years. Ninety five per cent are unilateral and 20% have metastasised at presentation, mainly to the lung and liver. Eighty per cent present with an abdominal mass, 25% with haematuria and approximately 30% with flank pain. Other features include failure to thrive and hemihypertrophy. It may be sporadic or familial, when Wilms' may be associated with aniridia, GU malformations and retardation (WAGR syndrome). The Wilms' tumour gene is found on chromosome 11.

Investigations of choice include IVU (renal pelvis distortion, hydronephrosis), USS and CT. Renal biopsy should be avoided. Treatment involves nephrectomy, chemotherapy (e.g. actinomycin E and radiotherapy which can be curative (80% five year survival). It is staged as follows:

Stage I: confined to kidney
Stage II: extrarenal spread but resectable
Stage III: extensive abdominal disease
Stage IV: distant metastases
Stage V: bilateral disease

2.17   **Answers: A C E**

Common side-effects of carbamazepine include nausea and vomiting, dizziness, drowsiness, headache, ataxia (phenytoin and clonazepam also have these effects), confusion and agitation (in the elderly), visual disturbances, anorexia, diarrhoea or constipation. A mild transient erythematous rash may occur in a large number of patients (this may need discontinuation of the drug if it worsens). Leukopenia and other blood disorders (thrombocytopenia, agranulocytosis and aplastic anaemia) are also recognised. Rickets is a known side-effect of phenytoin and phenobarbitone and transient hair loss is typical of sodium valproate.

2.18   **Answer: D**

A normal 18-month-old child can build a tower of 3–4 bricks and enjoys looking at books, turning the pages 2–3 at a time. They will spontaneously straight scribble holding the pen in a palmar grip (the tripod grip not developing until about three years of age). The ability to copy a straight line begins to develop just after 18 months with 90% of children achieving it by three years, while the ability to copy a circle develops after two years with 75% of children achieving it by three years.

2.19 **Answers: A B C D E**

A prolonged neonatal jaundice due to a conjugated hyperbilirubinaemia is a known presenting feature of cystic fibrosis and should be investigated. However a sweat test may be difficult to obtain from neonates, so alternative tests may be necessary (e.g. immune reactive trypsin). Any child with failure to thrive or short stature, especially if associated with respiratory or gastro-intestinal symptoms should also be investigated for cystic fibrosis. Pancreatic enzyme and dietary supplements are needed and may have to be increased when the child is ill (overnight tube feeding may be of benefit). Chest infections are common and cause progressive lung damage (i.e. bronchiectasis). The usual pathogens isolated are *Haemophilus influenzae*, *S. aureus*, Klebsiella and Pseudomonas. Treatment includes chest physiotherapy, i.v. antibiotics and nebulised bronchodilators.

2.20 **Answers: A C**

Common side-effects of clonazepam are somnolence (and paradoxical hyperactivity), muscle hypotonia, fatigue, dizziness, co-ordination disturbances and hypersalivation in infancy. Rarer side-effects include blood disorders and abnormal liver function. Acne occurs with phenytoin and nystagmus with overdose. Reversible leukopenia is more typical of carbamazepine.

2.21 **Answers: B C**

Roseola infantum is a common disease of infancy. It is commonly due to human herpes virus type 6 (herpes virus type 7 is also a likely pathogen). It has an incubation period of approximately 5–15 days, then typically presents with a high fever for 3–4 days which subsides as a fine maculopapular rash developing initially on the torso, before becoming widespread. It resolves in 2–3 days.

Human parvovirus type B19 is the cause of '5th disease', which is also known as the 'slapped cheek' syndrome and erythema infectiosum. Roseola infantum is also known as '6th disease' and its only significant complication is febrile convulsions. Measles and chickenpox are associated with pneumonia.

2.22 **Answers: A C**

Soto's syndrome (cerebral gigantism), Klinefelter's syndrome and Marfan's syndrome are all associated with tall stature.

2.23   **Answers: A B C**

Homocystinuria is a metabolic disorder associated with tall stature. Endocrine disorders resulting in tall stature include hyperthyroidism, precocious puberty and growth hormone excess (pituitary gigantism). Endocrine disorders resulting in short stature include pseudohypoparathyroidism, growth hormone deficiency, hypopituitarism, hypothyroidism and Cushing's disease.

2.24   **Answers: A B C D E**

Many infants who are acutely unwell (e.g. infection or electrolyte imbalance) will be apathetic and floppy on presentation. Werdnig–Hoffmann disease is also known as 'infantile spinal muscular atrophy' and classical features of Prader–Willi syndrome include hypotonia, hypogonadism and obesity.

2.25   **Answers: A C D E**

Cystic fibrosis is an autosomal recessive disorder and affects approximately 1 in 2000 live births in the UK. Presenting features include meconium ileus, recurrent respiratory infection, failure to thrive, loose stools, steatorrhoea and malabsorption. Other associated features include rectal prolapse, short stature, delayed puberty, diabetes mellitus, chronic sinusitis and nasal polyps.

2.26   **Answers: A D E**

Live attenuated vaccines include measles, mumps, rubella, BCG and the oral poliomyelitis vaccine (Sabin–OPV). They will provoke a cell-mediated response. Vaccines comprising inactivated organisms include pertussis and Salk (poliomyelitis–IPV), whereas vaccinations to tetanus and diphtheria comprise inactivated toxins. Both groups stimulate a primary response of antibody or antitoxin IgM and a secondary response of IgG. Hib is a component vaccine and stimulates an antibody IgM primary response.

2.27   **Answers: A B C**

Ninety five per cent of children with cystic fibrosis have pancreatic insufficiency that results in steatorrhoea and fat-soluble vitamin (A, D, E & K) deficiency requiring supplementation. Consequently treated children often have excellent appetites!, although undiagnosed, non-compliant or unwell children are often anorexic.

The investigation of choice is the sweat test, to confirm the diagnosis three tests should be abnormal (i.e. sweat sodium > 70 mmol/l). Cystic fibrosis is a Caucasian disorder, it has a lower incidence in Afro-Caribbeans and is very rare in the Chinese. Cystic fibrosis causes male infertility but not impotence.

2.28   **Answers: C D E**

Cromoglycate is ineffective in the treatment of acute asthma but is a useful prophylactic agent. Inhalers deliver less than 5% of the drug to the lungs and even nebulisers only deliver less than 10%. Aminophylline can be used in the management of an acute attack, however the loading dose should be omitted if the child is already on oral theophylline and ideally a drug level should be measured before the infusion is commenced.

Regular inhaled low dose steroids do not result in growth retardation. The incidence of oral candidiasis can be reduced if steroids are inhaled via a spacer device and rinsing the mouth afterwards reduces the risk further.

2.29   **Answers: A B D**

Conditions that may result in a false-positive sweat test include Addison's disease, hypothyroidism, nephrogenic diabetes insipidus, glucose-6-phosphatase deficiency, mucopolysaccharidosis and ecto-dermal dysplasia. Bronchiectasis is a clinical feature of cystic fibrosis, but will not cause a positive sweat test *per se.*

2.30   **Answers: A B D**

A normal 3-year-old child can imitate a three brick bridge and can build an eight brick tower with increasing confidence from about two years. They typically hold a pen with either a mature or tripod grip and can copy a straight line or a circle. Between 3–4 years they can copy a '+' and from four years will copy a square. They are unable to draw a man of six parts until about five years of age.

2.31   **Answers: A D E**

Part III of the 1993 Education Act is the UK legislation dealing with special educational needs (SEN); it replaces the 1981 Education Act. Its emphasis is on the earliest possible identification of SEN, including pre-school children and the importance of partnership between parents, children, schools, local education authorities (LEAs) and any other involved agencies. It aims to teach a wide and balanced curriculum, including the National Curriculum and most children with SEN, including those with statements, will have their needs met in mainstream schools. Statements of SEN should be made and reviewed annually.

A child has a learning difficulty if he or she has a significantly greater difficulty in learning than the majority of children the same age or has a disability which either prevents or hinders the child from making use of educational facilities of a kind provided for children of the same age in schools within the area of the LEA. Special educational provision includes any educational provision that is additional to or different from that provided by mainstream schools for a child over two years or any educational provision given to a child under two.

2.32   **Answers: A D**

Accidents are the single largest cause of death in children between one and 14 years and are responsible for approximately a third of all childhood deaths. Falls are the commonest accident, however road accidents (< 5% of all accidents) are the commonest fatal accident accounting for about 50% of accidental deaths.

Approximately 15% of all children per year attend A&E because of an accidental injury, the majority of these are boys aged 5–8 years from social classes IV and V.

2.33   **Answers: A C D**

Rhesus incompatibility is an iso-immune haemolytic disorder and G-6-PD deficiency also causes haemolysis. Consequently both result in an unconjugated hyperbilirubinaemia. Choledochal cysts and extrahepatic biliary atresia, on the other hand cause conjugated hyperbilirubinaemia, whereas hypothyroidism can cause both.

2.34   **Answers: B C E**

Primary prevention is aimed at preventing the 'accident' from happening and includes speed limits, stair gates, teaching road safety and child proof catches on cupboards.

Secondary prevention aims to prevent injury should the 'accident' happen. Examples of secondary prevention include cycling helmets, seat belts, smoke alarms and fire extinguishers kept in the house. N.B. Child resistant lids are a form of primary prevention as they prevent the child from reaching the drug, however blister packs for prescription drugs merely limit the number of a tablets a child can get at in a given time and are therefore a form of secondary prevention.

Tertiary prevention aims to limit the impact of an injury once the 'accident' has happened and includes teaching parents first aid skills and providing good access to the emergency services.

2.35   **Answers: A B D**

2.36   **Answers: A D E**

Bilirubin toxicity is caused by free unconjugated bilirubin that is lipid soluble and therefore readily crosses brain cell membranes. Kernicterus is rare in term infants if the serum bilirubin does not exceed 380 mmol/l, however premature infants or those with sepsis, hypoxia or acidosis may be affected at much lower levels. Symptoms include poor feeding, irritability, hypertonicity, opisthotonus, high-pitched cry, apnoea and convulsions.

Treatment involves phototherapy using a narrow spectrum blue light of wavelength 450–475 nm, this causes photo-isomerization and photo-oxidation of bilirubin to less lipophilic pigments. Management should also include ensuring adequate hydration and possible exchange transfusion. If the baby survives, long-term sequelae include choreoathetoid cerebral palsy, high frequency nerve deafness, paralysis of upward gaze and mental retardation.

2.37   **Answers: A B E**

The Dubowitz system is a system for estimating the gestational age of neonates from 26 to 44 weeks. It includes various neurological criteria (e.g. posture, head lag) and physical (or external) criteria which include: presence of oedema; skin texture; skin colour (not crying); skin opacity (trunk); lanugo (over back); plantar creases; nipple formation; breast size; ear form and firmness; and development of genitalia (i.e. presence of testes in scrotum).

2.38   **Answers: A B C D**

Features of congenital rubella syndrome include deafness, eye defects (microphthalmia, cataract, retinopathy and glaucoma), cardiac defects (patent ductus arteriosus, atrial septal defect and pulmonary stenosis), cerebral palsy, microcephaly, mental retardation and osteitis. Saddle nose is a feature of congenital syphilis.

2.39   **Answers: A B C**

Infants born to poorly controlled diabetic mothers may have sacral agenesis, hypomagnesaemia, hypocalcaemia, polycythaemia and Erb's palsy secondary to the increased risk of shoulder dystocia.

2.40   **Answers: A B C D E**

All are safe to use during breast-feeding, however thyroxine may interfere with neonatal screening for hypothyroidism.

2.41   **Answers: A C D E**

Nose picking is the most common cause of epistaxis in children and is usually from blood vessels on the nasal septum (Little's area). Other common causes include upper respiratory tract infections, atrophic rhinitis and foreign bodies. Rarer causes include bleeding disorders and tumours of the nose and sinuses. Hypertension is a common cause of epistaxis in adults, but is rare in children.

2.42   **Answer: A**

Before adoption proceeds informed consent from both natural parents (or mother if the child is illegitimate) is desirable. However, it is not needed if they cannot be found, are incapable of agreeing, have abandoned or neglected the child, have persistently ill-treated the child and are unlikely ever to be able to look after the child adequately. Applicants wanting to adopt a child must be aged 21 or more and adoption is arranged through registered agencies. The child must live with the adoptive parents for three months before the order is finalised, at which time all rights and responsibilities pass to the adoptive parents irreversibly. The original parents have no right of access.

The adopted child takes on the nationality of his adoptive parents and has no claim to maintenance or inheritance from his original parent(s). At age 18 years an adopted child is entitled to his original birth certificate.

2.43   **Answers: C D E**

Short-term fostering is usually less than six months, if a longer placement is required then adoption should be considered. Long-term fostering is preferred for older children, whereas adoption is more appropriate for younger children.

Fostering is more likely to be successful if there are children of a similar age in the placement family. There is usually a limit of three foster children per family, however more may be fostered if they are all siblings. All children in long-term foster care require a six monthly medical examination and the GP has a vital role in co-ordinating services and ensuring continuing medical care.

2.44   **Answers: C D E**

There are 20 deciduous or 'milk' teeth and 32 permanent teeth (including four wisdom teeth). Teething may cause irritability, excessive salivation and a flushed appearance, but there is no fever. The first tooth to appear is generally a lower central incisor. Children do not have the hand-eye co-ordination to clean their teeth adequately until about 8–10 years of age, therefore parents should re-brush their children's teeth at least once a day. Thumb sucking may result in malocclusion and requires an orthodontic assessment.

2.45   **Answer: B**

Aerosol inhalers are appropriate for children over ten years of age, however if their technique is poor, then a spacer device, which allows inhaled drugs to be given adequately at any age, may be appropriate. A plastic coffee cup makes an excellent homemade 'back-up' spacer device by simply making a small hole in the base for the inhaler and then placing the rim firmly over the child's mouth and nose while the metered dose is given. Dry powder inhalers are suitable for a child over five years and oral salbutamol syrup is often prescribed in primary care for the treatment of infants and toddlers, although an inhaler plus spacer device may be more beneficial.

2.46   **Answers: A C**

Infants with a UTI may present with vomiting, irritability and feeding problems. Between 2–5 years abdominal pain, fever, dysuria and frequency are classic, whereas schoolchildren have the more adult picture of dysuria, frequency, haematuria, loin pain and usually no fever. Vesico-ureteric reflux is found in approximately 35% of children with a UTI. There is significant risk of progressive renal damage in the under fives, thus prompt diagnosis and treatment is essential in children who should be investigated during or after their first UTI.

Bacteria multiply rapidly at room temperature and should be 'plated' within one hour of collection. However, if this is not possible they may be refrigerated for up to 24 hours. Pyuria occurs in 50% of UTIs, however there are other causes of pyuria including fever due to other causes, trauma, some drugs (e.g. diuretics), calculi and renal TB.

2.47   **Answers: B C D**

Sudden infant death syndrome (SIDS) is defined as death of an infant or young child which is unexpected by history and in whom a thorough post mortem fails to reveal an adequate explanation. The incidence varies worldwide with marked seasonal variation (increased in winter months) and is the leading cause of death in infants over one week of age.

Risk factors include male sex, multiple birth, LBW babies, associated respiratory infection, bottle feeding, social classes IV and V and the prone sleeping position (the supine position helps reduce the risk). A history of a sibling dying of SIDS increases the risk ten-fold, whereas maternal substance abuse increases the risk thirty-fold.

Management involves support and reassuring the parents they are not to blame. The need for a post mortem should be explained and if a twin, the sibling should be investigated and observed. The GP should visit the same day and follow up regularly over the next few weeks as once the acute shock is over, depression may ensue.

2.48   **Answers: C E**

Trimethoprim is usually the best first-line antibiotic, as *E. coli* (responsible for 80% of UTIs) is often resistant to amoxycillin. Augmentin, nitrofurantoin and cephalosporins are also useful. Trimethoprim and nitrofurantoin are often used as prophylaxis in children with vesico-ureteric reflux (VUR), and are effective when given once daily.

Prevention of UTIs includes the avoidance of constipation, ensuring the bladder is completely empty after voiding and wiping in a front-to-back direction. If there is no evidence of chronic pyelonephritis then treatment of asymptomatic bacteriuria is not recommended as it may allow a virulent strain to re-infect with the elimination of an avirulent one. Surgery may be necessary if the UTIs are secondary to calculi, obstruction or severe VUR.

2.49   **Answers: A B C D E**

2.50   **Answers: C D E**

Routine screening of all children for VUR does not fulfil Wilson and Jungner's criteria for cost-effectiveness. However, it is vital to investigate all children presenting with a UTI as approximately 35% will have VUR and about 35% of these go on to develop renal scarring which is the most important cause of renal hypertension and chronic renal failure in childhood. A micturating cysto-urethrogram is the diagnostic investigation of choice with renal growth and morphology being monitored by serial USS.

VUR is graded as follows:

    Grade I: reflux into lower end of ureter without dilatation
    Grade II: urine refluxes into the kidney on micturition only
    Grade III: reflux enters kidney during both bladder filling and
                 voiding
    Grade IV: reflux with dilatation of the ureter or renal pelvis

Management of grade IV VUR is debatable and should be referred for a urological opinion. Conservative medical management may be all that is required, however surgical re-implantation of the ureters or submucosal Teflon injections are alternatives.

2.51   **Answers: A D**
Scabies is caused by the *Sarcoptes scabiei* mite which burrows into the skin to lay eggs. Typical sites include the interdigital webs and flexor aspects of the wrists of older children and adults, however, the face and scalps of infants are often involved as well.

Sarcoptes scabiei is transmitted by close contact and has an incubation period of 2–4 weeks. Therefore, the whole family must be treated with gamma benzene hexachloride lotion on two occasions, seven days apart to ensure eradication. Clothing and bedding should be decontaminated by hot washing.

Pruritus, which is usually worse at night, is due to sensitisation and persists for 4–6 weeks post eradication. Symptomatic measures such as calamine lotion or antihistamine should be tried and further re-treatment avoided as this will lead to irritant dermatitis and resistance.

2.52   **Answers: A B C D**
Orthopaedic complications of obesity include Blount's disease and slipped femoral epiphyses. All obese healthy children are tall for their age with advanced bone age. If an obese child is short for their age it is important to exclude hypothyroidism, growth hormone deficiency, Cushing's, Down's and Prader–Willi syndromes.

2.53   **Answers: B E**
Cerebral palsy is a disorder of posture and movement resulting from a non-progressive lesion of the developing brain before or during the neonatal period. The expression of the lesion changes as the brain matures. It has a prevalence of 2.5 in 1000. Mental handicap occurs in < 50% of children. Other associated disabilities include visual (25%), language (90%) and hearing loss (25%).

The importance of various causes of cerebral palsy is controversial. Perinatal insult is now thought to be less important as an aetiological factor. Other causes include cryptogenic (35%), genetic (20%), postnatal disease e.g. meningitis (20%) and intra-uterine infection, irradiation or drug induced damage (5%).

Diagnosis of cerebral palsy under six months may be difficult unless it is severe. Similarly mild cases may only present with delayed developmental milestones or clumsiness.

2.54   **Answers: A D E**
The ketogenic diet is beneficial in some children with intractable seizures, however it is unpalatable and difficult to enforce. Protective helmets should be worn while cycling, however cycling (like swimming) must be supervised and busy/open roads avoided. It is also important that restrictions are kept to a minimum and education in normal schools the goal, with teachers kept informed about progress and drug treatment. In a small number of children with refractory epilepsy, surgery may give good results.

2.55   **Answers: B C D**
In spastic diplegia the legs are more severely affected than the arms; in spastic hemiplegia there is asymmetrical tone and reduced spontaneous movements on the affected side (arm relatively weaker than leg) with the limbs on the affected side being smaller, colder and spastic – although almost all children are usually walking by school age. Spastic hemiplegia may result from an infarct of the cortex or internal capsule and only about 30% have an IQ less than 70.

2.56   **Answers: A B C D E**

2.57   **Answers: A B D E**
Hirschsprung's disease presents with constipation. It is due to a congenital absence of intestinal autonomic ganglion cells of the Auerbach and Messier plexus and is also associated with hypertrophy of extrinsic autonomic nerves.
Causes of constipation include a low fibre diet, over-enthusiastic potty training, anal fissures, anal trauma (e.g. post operative, abuse), medication, dehydration, hypercalcaemia, hypothyroidism and spinal disorders (e.g. spina bifida).

2.58   **Answers: B C D E**
Phenylketonuria is an autosomal recessive condition with an incidence of 1:7000 in the UK. A heel prick blood test (the so-called Guthrie test) at day six looks for congenital hypothyroidism and can also detect elevated levels of phenylalanine. Phenylketonuria is associated with infantile spasms and will result in mental retardation if the diagnosis is delayed and dietary restrictions not enforced. These restrictions should be continued until the child is at least ten years old and ideally until adulthood. However, dietary restrictions should always be reinstated before conception and maintained throughout the pregnancy to improve outcome, as genetically normal babies may be affected antenatally by the elevated levels of phenylalanine in the maternal circulation.

2.59   **Answer: B**

Neither HIV nor AIDS are notifiable diseases. The risk of vertical transmission in Europe is between 13–25% and has been shown to be decreased by Caesarian section and antiviral drugs in pregnancy; although this figure is much higher in Africa. Testing neonates for the presence of HIV antibodies is not helpful in excluding a congenital infection because of the transmission of maternal antibodies. However, P24 antigen and polymerase chain reaction are of use.

Although the risk of transmission via breast milk is small, where safe alternatives are available breast-feeding should be avoided. However, in developing countries the risks of breast-feeding are far outweighed by the alternatives and should therefore be encouraged. N.B. HIV is a positive indication for *Pneumococcus* vaccination.

2.60   **Answers: B C D E**

1. *Advise the parents of a 10-year-old boy with normally well-controlled insulin dependent diabetes who develops a febrile illness.*

Infections, especially with fever, may lead to the loss of diabetic control and are a common cause of diabetic ketoacidosis, however, there is no evidence that diabetic patients with good control are more prone to infections than normal subjects. Therefore, it is appropriate to give the usual advice for the management of any febrile illness e.g. regular paracetamol to control the fever, encourage oral fluids to avoid dehydration, investigate the cause of the fever as clinically indicated and prescribe antibiotics if clinically appropriate.

In the case of diabetics the parents should be warned that their child may need to increase his dose of insulin by up to 25% in the presence of an infection. Therefore more frequent blood sugar monitoring is required for the duration of the illness with appropriate dose adjustment of the usual QDS injections. A normal diet should be encouraged and parents should be warned never to omit an insulin dose even if the child becomes clinically nauseated and unable to eat. Parents should check urine for ketones.

If diarrhoea and vomiting develops or glucose control is in danger of compromise, the parents should be advised to seek urgent medical help and possible hospital admission. Once the illness has settled the child may return to their normal insulin regime with the usual follow-up with the diabetic nurse.

2. *What are the characteristics of a child with a febrile convulsion that would suggest an increased risk of developing epilepsy?*

After a simple febrile convulsion 2% of children develop epilepsy which is no greater than the background risk. 10% of children with a previous neurological abnormality develop epilepsy after a febrile convulsion.

The risk of epilepsy is doubled after a complex febrile convulsion which accounts for 20% of all febrile convulsions.

A convulsion is described as complex if it:
- is focal
- lasts for more than 15 minutes
- the child has more than one convulsion per febrile illness
- the child is left with a residual neurological deficit

There is an increased risk if the febrile convulsion is secondary to meningitis or encephalitis. There is a 95% risk if the child has a family history of epilepsy.

Five per cent of epileptics have other secondary risk factors including:
- Perinatal factors (e.g. trauma, hypoxia, jaundice); cerebral tumours and malformations (vascular, neurofibroma, tuberous sclerosis, hydrocephalus)

3.   *How would you prevent the spread of head lice? Discuss methods of eradication.*

Prevention

- Avoid sharing combs/hair brushes etc.
- Avoid direct contact
- Hot wash clothes/linen that are infested
- Clean brushes etc.
- Routine hair checks at school
- Treat all close contacts e.g. other family members

Treatment

- **Malathion** 0.5% lotion applied to the hair overnight (the shampoo is generally not helpful as it is diluted and has only a brief contact with the hair). NB. Aqueous formulas are preferred in asthmatic and small children to avoid the alcoholic fumes however this is a second line treatment as it no longer ensures the death of the eggs.
- **Permethrin** (Pyrethriods) kills both eggs and lice and needs only a 10 minute application. NB. Lice have developed a low level of resistance therefore rotation of products is necessary to help prevent spread of resistant strains.
- After applying the above a 'nit' comb should be used to remove the eggs (long hair needs an application of diluted (1:1) vinegar or lemon juice before combing to help break down the attachment of nits to the hair shaft).
- If resistance is a problem, shaving may be acceptable to some boys.

4.   ***A seven-week-old baby has become inconsolable every evening for the last twelve days. What are the possible diagnoses and how would you manage this case?***

Differential diagnosis

- Hunger, boredom, tiredness, colic, wet nappy, early teething or other discomfort
- It is important to exclude a pathological cause e.g. infections, intermittent reducible hernia, cows' milk protein allergy and child abuse.

History

- Take a full history i.e. is the crying normal or abnormal, how long does it last and what is the pattern of the crying?
- Is it associated with feeding (increased or decreased milk delivery, mouth lesions, nasal obstruction)?
- Is it an established pattern due to stresses within the family (i.e. neglect, unhappiness, inappropriate handling or a difficult temperament)?
- Does the child appear in discomfort, hungry etc.?

Examination

- Perform a full examination including mouth and abdomen. Does the baby draw up its legs when crying?
- Look for signs specifically of injury or neglect
- Assess any developmental delay

Management

- Treat any pathological cause, but if none can be found appropriate management includes listening sympathetically, being supportive and comforting, recommending simple measures such as winding the child after feeding, carrying in a sling and advice on ways to stimulate the child such as sitting them up so they can see and taking them on 'walks'.
- Ensure the parents have realistic expectations of the child and recommend day nursery or family centre for respite.
- Ongoing support may be necessary as a lifeline to those without family backup e.g. Health Visitor, baby groups etc.
- Consider respite or admission if the child is 'at risk' or the parents are exhausted.

5.   What are the problems encountered with distraction hearing tests?

- Distraction hearing tests have a very low sensitivity and low specificity
- The test requires trained staff and is performed on children from six to 18 months of age. The child must be able to sit upright without support and have good head control and the test is therefore useless in children with gross motor developmental delay.
- Transient conductive hearing loss in a child with an upper respiratory tract infection or acute otitis media etc. can result in a temporary positive result, thus requiring the test to be repeated once the child has recovered.
- The tester should avoid wearing loud jewellery and particularly strong perfume or aftershave which may be detected by deaf children and will also result in false positives.
- False negatives can occur if the room is not soundproof, if there are creaking floor boards and poor lighting which casts shadows.

6.   How would you assess a five-year-old boy whose mother feels he is excessively 'clumsy' and has poor writing skills? Outline the general management plan.

Clumsiness may be regarded in any child, of whatever chronological age, whose general abilities are for example approximately 7 years old, but whose motor co-ordination skills are out of proportion at e.g. 4–5 years. They may also have other associated learning difficulties and are at risk of developing secondary emotional problems born from frustration or social isolation etc. The motor difficulties may be one or a combination of large movements (e.g. balance), hand-eye co-ordination, fine motor skills. The term is a vague one and doesn't indicate an aetiology, however this is important to establish as it will affect both the management and the prognosis.

History

- What does the mother mean by clumsy, is it acute or chronic, is it situation specific?
- Obtaining a school report may be helpful, are they concerned?
- A developmental history is also useful. Does he have frequent falls and poor balance; can he dress and feed himself; does he have a speech disorder, learning difficulties or any behavioural problems?

- Past medical history including antenatal, delivery, SCBU etc., and any hospital admissions.
- Family history: were his siblings or even his parents described as clumsy?
- Social history: assess the family dynamics and assess the possibility of physical/emotional abuse or neglect.

Examination

- This should include a full medical examination especially looking for signs of hyper-activity and emotional immaturity.
- A neurological examination to detect signs of mild cerebral palsy or cerebellar abnormalities. Any asymmetry of reflexes should be checked and look for any hypo/hypertonia.
- A gross motor developmental examination would include standing on one leg assessing the gait and seeing if they can hop, skip, kick a ball and walk heel to toe.
- A fine motor examination would include brick building, bead threading, finger thumb opposition in fast sequence, pencil grasp, writing skills and the ability to draw a man.
- The vision (and hearing) should also be tested.

Management

- Any appropriate further investigations should be performed depending on clinical findings e.g. cerebral palsy
- Once the cause has been identified (i.e. normal for the boy/family, hyperactive, mild CP or a specific motor problem) then the severity should be assessed. If it is mild will he cope in the main stream schools or if it is severe, will he need statementing?
- Advise the parents not to criticise the child and reassure him that he is not dull, careless or stupid.
- Emphasise the things he is good at, for example swimming, horse riding.
- Training is important as once a motor skill is learnt it is retained (cognitive) and talking through procedures may help i.e. in a graded series of steps.
- Involve the occupational therapist and physiotherapist (also parents, teachers and child psychologists) in the treatment plan.
- Stress that things should improve or that mild clumsiness is common and not often a significant handicap.
- If at all concerned refer to either the community paediatrician in a multi-disciplinary team, or a hospital specialist as appropriate.

7. **What are the symptoms and signs of a complex partial seizure (temporal lobe) in a school age child? Make a list of possible differential diagnoses.**

- The child may stare or have automatisms i.e. purposeless organised movement such as lip smacking, head turning and limb movements
- An aura may occur e.g. hallucinations (smell, taste, vision, abdominal pain, déjà vu)
- Altered consciousness is common, but this may not be obvious or accompanied by collapse
- Specific learning difficulties, mental handicap and behavioural problems occur more commonly than in other types of epilepsy
- They may have associated autonomic phenomenon (pallor/flushing) or facial asymmetry
- They may have mood changes or collapse
- There may be post-ictal confusion
- It usually lasts approximately 10 seconds
- Spike waves may be seen in the temporal lobe on EEG, particularly when the child is sleep deprived

Differential diagnosis

- Other atypical forms of epilepsy
- Drug or alcohol abuse
- Munchausen's syndrome or other psychiatric disorder
- Tics
- Migraines
- Arrhythmias
- Masturbation

8a. **List valid indications for performing a circumcision.**

- Religious/cultural
- Recurrent balanitis
- Phimosis (with scarring of foreskin) leading to urinary retention
- 'Ballooning' with post micturition dribbling
- Paraphimosis (forcible retraction leading to trapping of the foreskin)
- Parental request

8b. ***The majority of circumcisions (excluding religious/cultural reasons) are not performed for preputial disease. Why is this the case?***

- People may be more aware of the likely decrease in risk of cancer of the penis and cervix and the decreased risk of urinary tract infection
- Referral for inappropriate circumcisions e.g. for a non retractile foreskin which is normal in 96% of boys at birth, 10% at five years and 1% at 17 years of age. Preputial adhesions generally resolve without treatment and may be caused by misguided attempts to retract.
- In 3–5-year-olds a tight rim proximal to the meatal orifice can be loosened with 0.5% hydrocortisone cream applied twice daily for a few days, rather than an immediate referral for circumcision.
- Children may be referred after a single attack of balanitis, which may well never recur
- Parents may be unaware of the morbidity and even mortality associated with circumcision
- Children may be referred for 'ballooning' which, if the only symptom, can be left alone

9. ***Write short notes on the Emergency Protection Order and obtaining consent for children under 16 years.***

The Children's Act of 1989 replaces the 'Place of Safety' order, which lasted 28 days, with the Emergency Protection Order (EPO). This lasts 8 days and is renewable for 7 days. Parental responsibility is transferred to the applicant for the period of the order, although parents can challenge it in court after 72 hours.

Applications can be made by any person. The court may direct the police to enter premises to enforce the order and may specify where the child is to be held and any medical or other assessments required.

The Children's Act of 1989 states that below 16 years the consent of the parent or guardian is required unless:
- Emergency treatment is required when consent by a person i.e. teacher/doctor who is '*in loco parentis*' is appropriate or acceptable.
- The child has given their own consent and the doctor considers the child is of sufficient understanding to make an informed decision about medical care (including contraception)

If a child under 16 refuses consent the doctor cannot proceed (even if the child is under a care order etc.) unless:

- He believes the child does not have sufficient understanding to make an informed decision
- A court has considered the child's objection and told the doctor to proceed

If a parent/parents of a child under 16 years refuse life saving treatment, a court can give consent.

10.   *What is the differential diagnosis of persistent jaundice in a one-month-old infant? List useful investigations.*

Differential diagnosis

- Prolonged physiological jaundice (especially if breast-feeding)
- Infection +/- dehydration e.g. hepatitis A,B,C CMV etc.
- Hepatic enzyme defect e.g. Gilbert's syndrome
- Increased haemolysis e.g. red cell defect (spherocytosis, G6PD deficiency)
- Obstructive e.g. extrahepatic biliary atresia
- Metabolic e.g. galactosaemia
- Endocrine e.g. hypothyroidism
- Cystic fibrosis
- Idiopathic hepatitis

Ideally all investigations should begin with a thorough 'history & examination'

- Ask about the antenatal period and birth – was the baby premature or in SCBU?
- How long has the baby been jaundiced? When did it start, is it getting better or worse, have they had any treatment in hospital, is the child well or sick, are they breast or bottle feeding?
- Drug history
- Family history (especially of jaundice)
- Assess the level of jaundice, whether the child is alert/happy or sick/lethargic
- Is the baby febrile/dehydrated?
- Perform a full examination, especially the gastro-intestinal system, looking for hepatomegaly and the central nervous system looking for signs of kernicterus (irritable, increased tone, opisthotonus, high pitched cry, apnoea and fits)

Investigations

- Rhesus and ABO blood groups of both mother and infant (?Coombs test) – not very relevant in a 1-month-old baby with persistent jaundice
- Full blood count, blood film, reticulocyte count
- Conjugated and unconjugated bilirubin
- LFTs (especially transaminase and ALP)
- Thyroid function test
- Septic screen
- Viral titres (hepatitis A&B, CMV, EBV, HIV) viral culture
- Hepatic ultrasound scan
- Red cell enzymes for galactosaemia
- α–1 antitrypsin and phenotype
- Plasma and urine amino acids
- Urine for reducing substance
- Liver biopsy looking for hepatitis/biliary atresia

CASE COMMENTARY ANSWERS: PAPER 2

CASE COMMENTARY 1

1. What is your initial management of Emma?

Your initial management should always be basic life support assessing airway, breathing, circulation and proceeding onto advanced life support if necessary. An ambulance should be summoned urgently and the receiving Emergency Department telephoned regarding her imminent arrival. If Emma is stable she may be put into the recovery position to avoid aspiration while waiting for help to arrive, but should be regularly reassessed to make sure her condition has not deteriorated.

If possible a more detailed history should be obtained from the parents e.g. was Emma hot when fitting? How long did it last? Was it focal or generalised? Do a full examination including a neurological assessment looking for signs of raised intracranial pressure, meningism and petechial rashes. Particularly look for a septic focus e.g. ears/throat and if available always measure a bedside blood glucose.

2. Give your differential diagnosis. What are the most appropriate investigations you would order?

Possible differential diagnoses include febrile convulsion, intracranial infection, septicaemia, head injury, epilepsy, hypoglycaemia and poisoning.

Appropriate investigations include:
- Core/peripheral temperature, bedside blood glucose and a formal laboratory glucose
- Urea and electrolytes, calcium, magnesium, liver function tests +/- metabolic screen
- Full blood count
- Cultures including MSU, blood and CSF (the latter only after excluding raised ICP)
- ESR, CRP
- +/- EEG
- CT scan or MRI (head)
- Consider a drug screen

3. What is the probable diagnosis?

The most likely diagnosis is a non-accidental overdose of insulin by mum (Munchausen-by-proxy).

4. What is the most important investigation now?

If possible, insulin levels should be measured at the time of documented hypoglycaemia to see if a correlation occurs. You then need to determine whether the hypoglycaemia is due to an exogenous source of insulin i.e. drug induced or endogenous e.g. secondary to an insulinoma. Insulin is synthesised as a pro-hormone 'pro-insulin', which undergoes proteolytic cleavage to yield insulin and c-peptide. Therefore in an insulinoma the levels of c-peptide would be markedly raised whereas secondary to injection they would be low or normal. Thus, measurement of c-peptide levels during hypoglycaemia should identify if it is due to injecting insulin. Observation of the child and her parents is also important, especially their attitude to Emma, her illness, staff and events occurring during her admission.

5. Outline the points to be made at the case conference and the possible ways this family can be helped?

Child protection is paramount as Munchausen-by-proxy is associated with a significant mortality. Emma has a number of risk factors which make non-accidental poisoning more likely in her case.

1. Deliberate poisoning is common in the under twos (accidental poisoning occurs commonly between two and four years of age)
2. Emma is an only child, ?poor parenting skills
3. Family crises (dad's recent illness/recent move leading to possible social isolation)
4. Mum is a nurse and therefore has a medical knowledge of drugs
5. Did Emma's mother have an opportunity to poison her while in hospital and was she present just before the subsequent three episodes?
6. Report parents' response to her illness and their relationship with their child

Emma should not be returned to the sole care of her mother/parents if this diagnosis is felt to be likely and this decision should also be discussed at the case conference with legal advice.

Possible strategies for helping Emma's family include keeping her parents informed and involved at all times and possibly teaching them cardio pulmonary resuscitation. Encourage them to draw on an extended family for support and make sure they are aware of other available sources of support e.g. individual psychotherapy or family therapy, family centres, family rights groups, self help groups and telephone help lines.

CASE COMMENTARY 2

1. What history, examination and investigations would be most appropriate at this stage to help diagnose and manage this problem?

A good history is the most important part of Sarah's assessment, starting with the pregnancy, was it planned? Were there any problems antenatally, with the delivery or in the immediate neonatal period? You need to assess the extent of the problem i.e. when did it start, the type and pattern of disturbance, the effect on the family, the parental expectations and responses and ploys already tried.

It is also important to exclude medical causes, consider:
1. Chronic illness e.g. asthma (nights disturbed by coughing/distress) obstructive sleep apnoea (snoring, upper respiratory tract infections, rhinitis) chronic serous otitis
2. Prematurity, isolation from mother leads to later parental separation anxiety
3. Special needs e.g. learning difficulties
4. Temperament, some children have a very low sensory threshold

It is also important to assess any social and environmental factors:
1. Maternal absences, depression, illness, marital difficulties, alcohol or drug abuse
2. Adequate housing i.e. noise/damp/heat/excessive light
3. In some cultures it is common for the baby to sleep in the parental bed

Examination will probably be normal, although you may find evidence of any medical cause mentioned above. There are no specific investigations, however, some may be required to exclude a particular medical cause from the differential diagnosis.

2. What problems might Sarah's parents have and how will they affect the situation?

Sleep disturbance should be taken very seriously as sleep deprivation can result in a number of physical and psychosocial problems, including irritability, poor work performance, curtailment of sexual and social life and family arguments which may lead to violence inflicted upon a partner or child.

Tiredness or irritability will be 'picked up' by the infant leading to increased difficulties settling. Mum's pregnancy may lead to a further rift between Sarah's parents that can increase maternal anxiety. The father may also suffer from spiralling stress if he feels his poor performance at work may result in redundancy and possible deterioration in finances. The behavioural problems in Sarah's sibling may be secondary to tiredness, over disciplining from anxious parents or generally inadequate parenting skills.

Sarah may be 'trained to stay awake' e.g. she may be rewarded with a drink, cuddle or story by crying or better still taken to her parents bed. If one or both of the parents refuse to adhere to your treatment regime, you have to consider the possibility of secondary gain e.g. avoiding sex.

3. What advice would you give the parents handling this sleep problem? What other help is available (night sedation is shown to be of no benefit)?

As with any behaviour modification programme it is first necessary to clarify the objectives with the parents. It is important to assure them that their daughter does not have a 'serious' medical problem, that their difficulties are common and can be helped. They must also understand the need for a 'combined' approach to changing behaviour emphasising the need for consistency. During the day ensure Sarah has plenty of exercise, fresh air, regular playtime, regular meals and individual time spent with her mum. At bedtime she needs a familiar routine (cueing technique).

- Consider a light supper instead of milk to stop night-time hunger
- Bath/warm drink/clean teeth
- Own bed (adequate bedding) and own room if possible
- Quiet play time (story/picture books)
- Cuddly toy or security blanket
- Adjust lighting (night light and effective curtains)
- Relaxing sounds e.g. lullaby, taped music, ticking clock

- Soothing/relaxing techniques to settle e.g. stroking, massage or rocking

During the night respond to crying by attending to the child, but limit attention to excluding physical problems e.g. wet nappy. Do not attend as soon as she wakes but wait until she cries (children often wake transiently). Gradually increase the time the child is left to cry before attending. You can check every 5–10 minutes, if she's still crying but with minimal interaction. Do not provide drinks cuddles or stories, do not change the lighting or even talk to the child. Repeat minimal relaxation techniques (music) and if the parent must sit with the child they should be 'boring' so take something else to do.

If the child comes into the parents' bed the child must be quietly returned until this behaviour stops. Success may be achieved through a gradual change in behaviour i.e. a child who won't normally settle until 11 p.m. should have their bedtime routing brought slowly forward from 10.30 p.m. to 10 p.m. Positive reinforcement is generally only useful in children over three years. If the child is prone to sleep walking it is vital to ensure house safety.

Drug therapy is not used first line, however it may be useful in 'breaking the cycle' of parental sleep deprivation that may lead to an inability to undertake behavioural approaches. It should be prescribed for short-term use only and if used in children, beware paradoxical hyperactivity. Other help may be obtained from the grandparents who may offer to take Sarah for a few nights to allow the parents, and indeed Sarah's sister, to catch up on some sleep. Agreeing on a rota regarding who will look after Sarah and who will sleep each night is also helpful. There are various manuals and pamphlets that offer good advice and are available from the health visitor and local libraries, telephone help lines are also useful. Early postnatal anticipation and guidance may prevent the establishment of long-term sleep difficulties in infants.

60 questions: time allowed 2 hours
Indicate your correct answers with a tick in the boxes provided

3.1 Acute lymphoblastic leukaemia (ALL)

❑ A accounts for 85% of all childhood leukaemia
❑ B commonly presents with bone and joint pain
❑ C is more common in girls
❑ D the presence of a B cell immunological surface membrane marker is associated with the best prognosis
❑ E Epstein–Barr virus is associated with an increased risk of developing leukaemia

3.2 With regard to spina bifida

❑ A spina bifida occulta is seen in 5–10% of all children's spines
❑ B Arnold–Chiari malformation is frequently associated with myelomeningocele
❑ C myelomeningocele characteristically causes spastic paraplegia of the lower limbs
❑ D meningocele has no neurological involvement
❑ E myelomeningocele is characteristically associated with incontinence of urine, but not of faeces

3.3 Signs of sexual abuse in children include

❑ A HIV infection
❑ B clitoromegaly
❑ C sexualised behaviour inappropriate for age
❑ D anal fissures
❑ E anal skin tags

3.4 With regard to paracetamol poisoning

❑ A serious hepatotoxicity is likely if the four hour serum level is > 200 mg/L
❑ B it should be treated with ipecacuanha if seen within four hours of ingestion
❑ C it may cause jaundice and liver tenderness within 48 hours
❑ D an overdose of > 50 mg/kg is clinically significant
❑ E oral methionine is the treatment of choice within the first eight hours

3.5   Congenital rubella is characteristically associated with

- ❏ A deafness with maternal infection at 10–16 weeks' gestation
- ❏ B retinopathy
- ❏ C hydrocephalus
- ❏ D polycythaemia
- ❏ E neonatal conjugated hyperbilirubinaemia

3.6   The following incubation periods are correct:

- ❏ A chickenpox: 2–5 days
- ❏ B measles: 7–14 days
- ❏ C glandular fever: 14–21 days
- ❏ D mumps: 12–31 days
- ❏ E rubella: 7–14 days

3.7   Infantile colic

- ❏ A characteristically presents with paroxysmal crying and 'pulling up' of the legs
- ❏ B peaks between three and six months
- ❏ C is due to cows' milk allergy
- ❏ D there is no effective medical treatment
- ❏ E may require hospital admission

3.8   Signs of severe acute asthma include

- ❏ A presence of a loud wheeze
- ❏ B being too breathless to eat
- ❏ C a heart rate between 100 and 140/min
- ❏ D a peak flow (PEFR) < 50% of predicted
- ❏ E a respiratory rate of > 50/min

3.9   With regard to cleft palate

- ❏ A it may cause hearing loss
- ❏ B all babies with cleft palate should be admitted to SCBU for NG feeding
- ❏ C it should be repaired at three months
- ❏ D speech generally recovers in approximately 75% of children
- ❏ E it is associated with maternal epilepsy

3.10   A normal 18-month-old child

❏ A   can help in simple household tasks
❏ B   can use a knife and fork
❏ C   can point to different parts of the body
❏ D   can follow simple directions
❏ E   uses sentences of 8–10 words

3.11   The prevalence of asthma is increased with

❏ A   female sex
❏ B   family history of eczema
❏ C   forceps delivery
❏ D   passive smoking during pregnancy
❏ E   urban dwellers

3.12   Epidemiology of asthma

❏ A   causes approximately 50 deaths per year in the UK
❏ B   the majority of deaths occur amongst 0–4 year olds
❏ C   asthma affects 2–5% of all children in the UK
❏ D   the prevalence has gradually been decreasing over the last 20 years.
❏ E   the mortality rate has gradually been decreasing over the last 10 years

3.13   A normal 3-year-old child

❏ A   can lace up his own shoes
❏ B   will play interactive games (e.g. tag) with other children
❏ C   is not yet capable of imaginary play
❏ D   is 'dry' by day, but seldom at night
❏ E   is able to dress themselves without supervision

3.14   With regard to immunisations

❑ A   the Hib vaccine was made part of the immunisation schedule
in 1982

❑ B   low dose diphtheria antitoxin is now given as a booster to
school leavers due to a Russian epidemic in 1991 caused by
poor immunisation coverage and decreased immunity in
adults

❑ C   it is worthwhile vaccinating susceptible contacts of patients
with rubella

❑ D   it is worthwhile vaccinating susceptible contacts of patients
with measles

❑ E   a Heaf test is often falsely positive for up to one month
following the MMR

3.15   The stepwise treatment of asthma involves

❑ A   step 2: the regular use of low dose inhaled steroids and
bronchodilators as required

❑ B   starting at 'step one' and gradually stepping up treatment until
an appropriate level is reached

❑ C   step 4: the regular use of high dose systemic steroids

❑ D   'stepping down' if control has been good for over three
months

❑ E   step 5: the addition of slow release xanthine, ± nebulised beta-
agonist, ± alternate day prednisolone, ± ipratropium or beta-
agonist subcutaneous infusion

3.16   Concerning cystic fibrosis

❑ A   the gene for cystic fibrosis is located on the long arm of
chromosome 7

❑ B   it may be diagnosed antenatally by chorionic villous biopsy

❑ C   the risk of two carriers having an affected child is 1 in 2

❑ D   it has a gene carrier rate of 1 in 40 of the Caucasian
population

❑ E   approximately 75–80% of cystic fibrosis gene mutations in the
UK are due to a deletion at delta F508

3.17 Urinary tract infection (UTI)

- ❏ A is commoner in boys in the first month of life
- ❏ B *E. coli* is responsible in approximately 80% of cases
- ❏ C most UTIs are haematogenous in origin in neonates
- ❏ D significant bacteriuria occurs with > 10^3 bacteria/ml
- ❏ E vesico-ureteric reflux (VUR) is found in approximately 35% of children with a UTI

3.18 Infantile spasms

- ❏ A are also known as 'salaam attacks'
- ❏ B onset is usually after nine months
- ❏ C characteristically involve 'drop attacks' secondary to brief myoclonus or atonia
- ❏ D the EEG characteristically shows hypsarrhythmia in approximately 66%
- ❏ E first-line treatment involves prednisolone or ACTH

3.19 Generalized 'absences'

- ❏ A are more common in girls
- ❏ B are associated with mental retardation
- ❏ C 30% go on to develop generalized tonic-clonic epilepsy
- ❏ D the EEG shows unilateral spike waves over Rolandic
- ❏ E first-line treatment is carbamazepine

3.20 Generalized tonic-clonic epilepsy

- ❏ A onset is generally after five years of age
- ❏ B is not associated with an aura
- ❏ C the EEG may be normal between seizures
- ❏ D after 15 years approximately 80% remain 'fit-free' off treatment
- ❏ E first-line treatment is carbamazepine

3.21 Cerebral palsy

- ❏ A is a contraindication to the pertussis vaccine
- ❏ B may be secondary to hypoglycaemia in the perinatal period
- ❏ C features include their lack of primitive reflexes
- ❏ D may be associated with impaired hearing
- ❏ E feeding difficulties arise from hypotonia

3.22   Chronic constipation

- ❏ A   often presents with diarrhoea
- ❏ B   is normal in breast-fed babies
- ❏ C   is frequently diet related
- ❏ D   is associated with Down's syndrome
- ❏ E   is defined as the infrequent passage of stools

3.23   Risk factors for physical abuse include

- ❏ A   having a stepfather
- ❏ B   recent parental divorce
- ❏ C   birth at 31 weeks' gestation
- ❏ D   a child aged between four and eight years
- ❏ E   grandparents living nearby

3.24   Pica

- ❏ A   is defined as 'eating of things that are not food'
- ❏ B   it is usually an isolated behaviour
- ❏ C   the 'mouthing' of objects seen at about eight months is a good example
- ❏ D   is associated with iron deficiency anaemia
- ❏ E   which does not respond to disciplinary approaches, may require referral to a community paediatrician

3.25   Concerning hyperkinetic syndrome (attention deficit disorder)

- ❏ A   there is a boy:girl ratio of 10:1
- ❏ B   it may be associated with lead poisoning
- ❏ C   it may be associated with food additives
- ❏ D   it has an incidence in the USA of 5–10%
- ❏ E   behavioural therapy is the mainstay of treatment

3.26   Non-accidental injury should be suspected if

- ❏ A   parents attend A&E immediately
- ❏ B   parents are over protective
- ❏ C   a fractured tibia is seen in a six-month-old infant
- ❏ D   the child has a depressed skull fracture
- ❏ E   the child has bilateral black eyes

3.27 Case conferences for child abuse

❏ A the Butler-Schloss report recommends that parents must always be invited to attend the case conference

❏ B should ideally be held during the Emergency Protection Order (EPO)

❏ C the GP should be invited to attend

❏ D have only the capacity to decide whether the child should be placed on the Child Protection Register

❏ E must be attended by a senior officer from the social services

3.28 Salicylate poisoning

❏ A can cause a respiratory alkalosis

❏ B can cause a metabolic acidosis

❏ C can cause hypoglycaemia

❏ D the child may be discharged if the four hour serum salicylate level is 800 mg/L

❏ E treatment may involve vitamin K and FFP

3.29 Features of Kawasaki syndrome include

❏ A generalised lymphadenopathy

❏ B fever typically lasting at least five days

❏ C urgent echocardiography is required to exclude coronary artery aneurysms

❏ D thrombocytopenia

❏ E generalised urticarial or morbilliform rash

3.30 Reye's syndrome

❏ A is acute encephalopathy with fatty degeneration of the liver, kidneys and pancreas

❏ B is associated with ibuprofen exposure in young children

❏ C usually presents before the age of two years

❏ D is commonly complicated by hypoglycaemia

❏ E ALT, AST and bilirubin are usually elevated

3.31   Fallot's tetralogy

☐ A   typically has a left to right shunt
☐ B   typically has a pansystolic murmur
☐ C   cyanotic spells may be prevented by treatment with beta-blockers
☐ D   has the characteristic chest X-ray (CXR) appearance of an 'egg lying on its side'
☐ E   together with transposition of the great arteries (TGA) are the two leading causes of cyanotic congenital heart disease

3.32   Coarctation of the aorta

☐ A   is associated with Turner's syndrome
☐ B   should always be surgically corrected
☐ C   there is classically hypertension in the lower limbs
☐ D   characteristically has a 'continuous machinery' murmur
☐ E   the classical 'rib-notching' can be seen on the neonatal chest X-ray

3.33   Congenital heart disease

☐ A   Down's syndrome is associated with an increased incidence of VSD and ASD
☐ B   has an incidence of approximately 8 per 10,000 live births
☐ C   an indomethacin infusion can be used to keep the ductus arteriosus patent until corrective surgery can be carried out.
☐ D   ventriculo-septal defect (VSD) is the commonest congenital heart defect
☐ E   the incidence of cyanotic congenital heart disease is approximately three times that of acyanotic lesions

3.34   Regarding torsion of the testis

☐ A   peak incidence is approximately ten years of age
☐ B   it may present with hip pain
☐ C   there is an increased incidence if the testis is high and lying in the horizontal position
☐ D   it must be confirmed by USS prior to surgical exploration
☐ E   it is associated with inguinal hernia

3.35 Features of a headache that would support the diagnosis of a simple migraine

☐ A preceded by transient visual field defects and micropsia
☐ B papilloedema
☐ C strabismus
☐ D diplopia
☐ E nystagmus

3.36 The following associations are correct:

☐ A Noonan's syndrome and hypertrophic cardiomyopathy
☐ B Turner's syndrome and a narrow carrying angle
☐ C Edward's syndrome and rocker bottom feet
☐ D Pierre Robin syndrome and macrognathia
☐ E Laurence–Moon–Biedl syndrome and night blindness

3.37 Features of nephrotic syndrome include

☐ A proteinuria, hypoalbuminaemia, generalised oedema and hyperlipidaemia
☐ B the commonest cause of idiopathic (primary) nephrotic syndrome is diffuse proliferative glomerulonephritis
☐ C a serum albumin of < 35 g/l
☐ D a high protein, no salt diet should be strictly adhered to
☐ E peak incidence is between two and five years of age

3.38 Tuberculin testing

☐ A traditionally involves an injection into the extensor surface of the left forearm
☐ B the Heaf test should ideally be read between 48 and 72 hours
☐ C a positive result occurs when the area of induration is > 5 mm
☐ D is negative if a 'Heaf grade 1'
☐ E induration > 15 mm requires further investigation and possible antituberculous chemotherapy

3.39   Down's syndrome

❑   A   is associated with an increased incidence of duodenal atresia
❑   B   is the single commonest cause of severe learning difficulty
❑   C   is associated with hypothyroidism
❑   D   trisomy 21 has a recurrence risk of 10%
❑   E   is associated with general hypertonia

3.40   Rickets

❑   A   is associated with epilepsy
❑   B   may be secondary to ulcerative colitis
❑   C   causes both genu valgum and genu varum
❑   D   vitamin D resistant rickets is an autosomal dominant condition
❑   E   is associated with swelling at the wrists and costochondral junctions

3.41   Iron deficiency anaemia

❑   A   is a common presentation of threadworm infestation
❑   B   the total iron binding capacity (TIBC) is decreased
❑   C   coeliac disease is a predisposing factor
❑   D   typically has a hypochromic microcytic blood film with target cells
❑   E   may be prevented by early introduction of cows' milk to the infant diet

3.42   Beta-thalassaemia

❑   A   typically has a hypochromic microcytic blood film with target cells
❑   B   is associated with an increased incidence in Burma
❑   C   total iron binding capacity (TIBC) is markedly reduced
❑   D   vaccination against pneumococcus is contraindicated
❑   E   management involves daily iron supplements

3.43   Sickle cell anaemia

❑   A   carriage of HBs occurs in approximately 10% of UK
          Afro-Caribbeans
❑   B   heterozygotes show hypochromia, target cells, Howell–Jolly
          bodies and occasional sickle cells on their blood film
❑   C   can be diagnosed antenatally
❑   D   homozygotes are at an increased risk of biliary colic
❑   E   painful crises develop from about six months of age in
          homozygotes

3.44   Haemophilia

❑   A   haemophilia B is an autosomal recessive disorder
❑   B   children with haemophilia A must never be given aspirin
❑   C   the prothrombin time is normal in both haemophilia A and B
❑   D   regular dental care is essential
❑   E   is associated with progressive joint destruction

**3.45   Regarding glucose-6-phosphate dehydrogenase (G6PD)
          deficiency**

❑   A   fava beans should be avoided in the African variant
❑   B   nitrofurantoin may precipitate acute haemolysis
❑   C   cefuroxime is safe to use
❑   D   the blood film shows Howell–Jolly bodies
❑   E   treatment may involve the use of methylene blue

3.46   Causes of generalised lymphadenopathy include

❑   A   sarcoidosis
❑   B   Kawasaki disease
❑   C   phenytoin therapy
❑   D   eczema herpeticum
❑   E   juvenile chronic arthritis

**3.47   Poor prognostic features of acute lymphoblastic leukaemia
          include**

❑   A   age < 2 years
❑   B   age > 10 years
❑   C   Caucasians
❑   D   male sex
❑   E   a presenting WCC > 20,000 mm^3

3.48   In chronic diarrhoea

❏   A   in the UK, cows' milk protein intolerance is the most common cause of chronic diarrhoea in infants under one year

❏   B   recognizable food in the stool suggests toddler diarrhoea

❏   C   flat mucosa devoid of villa on a jejunal biopsy is diagnostic of coeliac disease

❏   D   coeliac disease most commonly presents between six and nine months of age

❏   E   ulcerative colitis is inherited in an autosomal recessive manner

3.49   Regarding tonsils and adenoids

❏   A   purulent follicular exudate is present only in bacterial tonsillitis

❏   B   a three day course of penicillin is adequate treatment for bacterial tonsillitis

❏   C   recurrent febrile convulsions associated with attacks of follicular tonsillitis are an indication for a tonsillectomy

❏   D   primary post-tonsillectomy haemorrhage is usually due to infection

❏   E   adenoidectomy is useful in the treatment of glue ear

3.50   In acute otitis media

❏   A   the most common causative organisms are viruses

❏   B   phenoxyethylpenicillin (penV) is the antibiotic of choice

❏   C   30% of children will have a residual middle ear effusion three months after an acute attack

❏   D   referral to an ENT surgeon should be considered for children having two or more attacks in one year

❏   E   there may be bullous formation on the eardrum

3.51   Appendicitis

❏   A   is rare in the under 5s ($< 2\%$)

❏   B   nearly 90% of cases present with perforation in under fives

❏   C   abdominal pain usually presents in the right iliac fossa

❏   D   differential diagnosis include mesenteric adenitis, urinary tract infection and diabetic ketoacidosis

❏   E   assessing the child's ability to 'hop' helps confirm the diagnosis

3.52   The role of the Health Visitor includes

❏   A   supervising the running of Immunisation Clinics
❏   B   reviewing every child under five years who has attended the A&E Department
❏   C   child health surveillance in all children under ten years of age
❏   D   taking over postnatal care from the midwife at three weeks of age
❏   E   responsibility for supervision of children in care

3.53   Language delay

❏   A   when severe, has an incidence of approximately 1 in 5000
❏   B   has an increased incidence amongst boys
❏   C   is associated with cleft palate
❏   D   the Reynals developmental language scale accurately assesses comprehension and expression
❏   E   has an increased incidence in large families

3.54   Inflammatory bowel disease

❏   A   both Crohn's and ulcerative colitis are associated with finger clubbing, anaemia, erythema nodosum and arthritis
❏   B   Crohn's disease has increased over the last 20–30 years and now affects about 5 per 10,000 individuals
❏   C   ulcerative colitis is characterised by inflammation of the whole thickness of the bowel wall, especially the terminal ileum and proximal colon
❏   D   the 'string sign', 'skip lesions' and 'rose thorn ulcers' are characteristically seen in Crohn's disease following a barium meal and follow through
❏   E   surgery is always required in the management of ulcerative colitis

3.55   Precocious puberty

❏   A   is defined as the onset of sexual maturation before ten years in a girl
❏   B   is associated with McCune–Albright syndrome
❏   C   results in an increased final height
❏   D   is commonly associated with intracranial tumours in boys
❏   E   is associated with coeliac disease

3.56 Anorexia nervosa

☐ A affects 1 in 250 girls between the ages of 15–18 years
☐ B primary amenorrhoea may be present
☐ C is associated with hyperkalaemia
☐ D has a mortality rate of 1%
☐ E is characterised by having a disturbed perception of body image

3.57 Low birth weight infants

☐ A premature infants are those born before 36 completed weeks' gestation
☐ B very low birth weight infants are those weighing < 2500 g
☐ C are characteristically associated with maternal diabetes
☐ D have an increased incidence of congenital malformations
☐ E babies who are small for gestational age may reflect maternal diabetes

3.58 Bow legs (genu varum)

☐ A are normal in infants and usually correct by five years of age
☐ B may be secondary to osteogenesis imperfecta
☐ C when due to 'medial tibial torsion', it is associated with bowing of the tibia which usually requires surgical correction
☐ D may be secondary to poliomyelitis
☐ E may be secondary to Osgood–Schlatter's disease

3.59 Ophthalmology

☐ A ophthalmia neonatorum is most commonly caused by *Neisseria gonorrhoeae*
☐ B Stevens–Johnson syndrome is associated with iritis
☐ C orbital cellulitis is commonly secondary to adjacent sinusitis
☐ D glaucoma may be associated with aniridia
☐ E intrauterine toxoplasmosis infection results in an increased incidence of cataracts

3.60   Investigation of recurrent UTI

❏   A   a micturating cysto-urethrogram (MCU) should be performed acutely to exclude vesico-ureteric reflux

❏   B   dimercaptosuccinic acid (DMSA) is used for detecting renal scarring

❏   C   diethylene triamine penta-acetic acid (DTPA) assesses differential function between both kidneys and between different areas of the same kidney

❏   D   all children less than one year should be investigated with an USS, DMSA and MCU after their first UTI

❏   E   children over six years require investigation with an AXR and USS only after their first UTI

SHORT NOTE QUESTIONS – PAPER 3

10 questions: time allowed 1 hour 30 minutes
Write short notes of the following subjects. Conciseness will be
beneficial. Lists are acceptable.

1. List the pros and cons in performing a splenectomy on a child with a hereditary spherocytosis. Outline your long-term management plan.

2. Discuss 'cyanotic breath holding' attacks. What advice would you give mother?

3. What features would make you suspect a non-accidental injury in a toddler with a periorbital bruise? What are the aims of a Child Protection Conference?

4. Write short notes on unilateral cryptorchidism.

5. What is cerebral palsy? Outline different methods of its classification.

6. An 11-month-old girl presents with a 7 hour history of screaming episodes approximately every 20 minutes appearing calm between attacks. Discuss your management of the most likely diagnosis.

7. What is the differential diagnosis of a 10-month-old child presenting with fresh blood on the surface of his stools. How would you manage this case?

8. Write short notes on school refusal versus truancy.

9. A toddler develops a febrile illness. On examination a murmur is heard on auscultation. What features imply it is not significant?

10a. What factors predispose to iron deficiency in the under two-year-olds?
10b. Is screening for iron deficiency beneficial and how would you go about it?

CASE COMMENTARIES – PAPER 3

Two questions: time allowed 1 hour 30 minutes
Read the following case history carefully. Then answer <u>all</u> the
questions below. Please start your answer on a separate page.

CASE COMMENTARY 1

Jane is an 18-month-old twin, at a recent home visit the health visitor was concerned to find her underweight, unable to walk and with severe nappy rash. Her sister however, was thriving and had been walking for two months. They were born at 32 weeks gestation and weighed 1.3 kg and 1.5 kg respectively. Jane developed respiratory distress syndrome shortly after birth requiring ventilation and a cranial ultrasound scan showed bilateral peri-ventricular haemorrhages with persisting right-sided parenchymal changes. Her sister progressed well and was allowed home early. They were followed up in Outpatients for eight months but then moved from the area and lost contact. All their immunisations are up to date.

Mother is 22 years old and a full time mum. Dad is 23 years old and works as a builder facing redundancy. They also have a 3-year-old son who was recently seen in the Accident and Emergency department with a greenstick fracture of his right wrist following a fall.

1. **Discuss the possible differential diagnosis and assess her failure to thrive.**

2. **Differentiate the various possible reasons for her inability to walk.**

3. **Outline methods of helping this family.**

CASE COMMENTARY 2

Chloe is 11 years old, she is complaining of an intermittent cough and decreased appetite. The cough started gradually approximately six months ago, it is worse when Chloe is distressed about something. It does not affect her sleep and is not exacerbated by exercise. Chloe has always been slim with a good appetite, however she has recently lost interest in food saying it makes her feel bloated. Her parents feel that she has lost weight. Chloe is normally fit and well, she is at the top of her class and particularly enjoys physical education. She also attends ballet classes after school. Her father is a company executive; he has frequent business trips abroad. Her mother is a part time lecturer at the local university and her younger sister is well.

On examination Chloe seemed shy, her height is on the 75th centile, however her weight is on the 25th centile. General examination is otherwise normal although she is pre-pubertal and has cool peripheries.

1.   Describe her cough and how you would investigate it.

2.   How would you investigate her poor appetite?

All investigations are normal; at review four weeks later she's eating even less and has lost 3 lbs in weight.

3.   What would you discuss with Chloe and her parents at this point?

4.   What strategies would you use to assist Chloe?

MULTIPLE CHOICE QUESTION PAPER 3 – ANSWERS

3.1 **Answers: A B**

Acute lymphoblastic leukaemia is the leading paediatric malignancy and accounts for 85% of all childhood leukaemias. The peak incidence is between 2–6 years, with boys being slightly more affected than girls (55% v. 45%). Common presenting features include sepsis, lethargy, pallor, bleeding, bruising, petechiae, skeletal pain secondary to leukaemic infiltration, lymphadenopathy and hepatosplenomegaly.

Investigations include a bone marrow aspiration and a blood film that reveals anaemia, thrombocytopenia and usually circulating blast cells. ALL is subdivided according to its immunological surface membrane markers, with 'common' having the best prognosis and 'B cell' the worst. Treatment involves ensuring good hydration, and allopurinol prior to chemotherapy in order to avoid renal impairment from urate stone formation. Epstein–Barr virus is associated with an increased incidence of developing Burkitt lymphoma.

3.2 **Answers: A B D**

Spina bifida occulta is seen in 5–10% of all children and is usually found incidentally on X-ray. In meningocele the dorsal laminae are absent with a skin-covered lesion containing only CSF without underlying neurological involvement.

Myelomeningocele is associated with neurological involvement. The neurological deficit depends on the level of the lesion, but double incontinence is the norm with paraplegia of the lower limbs. Both spastic and flaccid paralyses are seen, but the latter is more typical. 90% of affected children develop a hydrocephalus, which is most commonly secondary to an Arnold–Chiari malformation.

3.3 **Answers: C D E**

There may be general signs of sexual abuse (e.g. superficial injuries, recurrent UTI); perineal signs (e.g. soreness, vaginal discharge); and behavioural signs (e.g. sexualised behaviour, depression, bedwetting, drug dependence).

Chlamydia and genital warts are the common sexually transmitted diseases (STDs) in child sex abuse. HIV infection in children is generally through vertical transmission. Anal fissures, skin tags, reflex dilatation and perianal bruising are also suspicious of, but not pathognomonic of sexual abuse.

3.4   **Answer: A**

Serious hepatotoxicity is likely if > 150 mg/kg is ingested or if the four hour serum level is > 200 mg/L. Inducing vomiting is no longer recommended due to the potential risks of aspiration, activated charcoal is preferred. Oral methionine can be used if the patient presents within ten hours but may be rendered ineffective if the patient is vomiting or charcoal has been given. Therefore, i.v. N-Acetylcysteine is recommended as first-line treatment of choice. Jaundice and liver tenderness characteristically occur after 48 hours.

3.5   **Answers: B E**

The fetus is most at risk in the first 16 weeks of gestation, with approximately 55% affected if maternal infection occurs in the first four weeks. Cataract is associated with infection at 8–9 weeks, deafness at 5–7 weeks (although may occur with 2nd trimester infection) and cardiac lesions at 5–10 weeks. Other features include purpura, jaundice, hepatosplenomegaly, microcephaly, microphthalmia, retinopathy, developmental delay, cerebral palsy and thrombocytopenia. Miscarriage or stillbirth may also occur.

3.6   **Answers: B D**

The characteristic incubation periods for the following conditions are: chickenpox (10–24 days); measles (7–14 days); glandular fever (30–50 days); mumps (12–31 days) and rubella (14–21 days).

3.7   **Answers: A D E**

Infantile colic characteristically presents with paroxysmal crying and 'pulling up' of the legs and rarely lasts beyond three months of age. There is no known cause and a child should only be labelled as having colic by exclusion of all other likely and dangerous diagnoses. Although there is no clinically effective treatment, the child may require a social admission to hospital to break the cycle of stressed mother and crying baby.

3.8   **Answers: B D E**

The British Thoracic Society guidelines define acute severe asthma as being: too breathless to talk; too breathless to feed; respirations > 50/min; pulse > 140/min and a PEFR < 50% predicted or best. Life-threatening features are defined as: PEFR < 33% predicted or best; cyanosis, a silent chest, or poor respiratory effort; fatigue or exhaustion; and agitation or decreased level of consciousness. Children with severe attacks may not appear distressed and assessment in the young may be difficult. Therefore the presence of any of the above features should alert the doctor.

3.9   **Answers: A D E**

Antiepileptics taken antenatally increase the incidence of cleft lip and palate. Cleft lip should be repaired at three months, but cleft palate repair should be between six months and one year. If surgery is performed during this time and the help of a speech therapist is enlisted, then speech has about a 75% chance of developing normally. Cleft palate may cause hearing loss due to the increased incidence of otitis media with effusion. Admission to SCBU should be avoided as this can hinder bonding. Special teats are available to use before surgical repair if feeding is problematical.

3.10   **Answers: A C D**

A normal 18-month-old child can help in simple household tasks, can point to different parts of the body and can follow simple commands (e.g. give me the ball). They can use a spoon, spilling little, but are unable to master a knife and fork. A child of 15 months to two years will generally be using simple two word combinations (e.g. want drink). By two years the child may have simple sentences of three or four words.

3.11   **Answers: B E**

The prevalence of asthma is increased with male sex, a personal or first-degree family history of atopy and amongst urban dwellers. Maternal smoking during pregnancy or passive smoking postnatally are also associated with an increased prevalence. Forceps delivery bears no relation to the risk of developing asthma, although a low birth weight is relevant.

3.12   **Answer: A**

Asthma affects > 10% of children and causes approximately 50 deaths per year in the UK. Most are teenagers with chronic severe asthma. The prevalence has been gradually increasing over the last 20 years. This may be due to increased parental awareness, pollution and changing infant feeding patterns. The mortality has however remained static.

3.13   **Answers: B E**

A normal 3-year-old is usually 'dry' both day and night. They can feed, wash and dress themselves without supervision, including donning shoes, but are unable to manage complex buckles or laces. They will interact with other children in both imaginary and non-imaginary play.

3.14   **Answers: B D**

The Hib vaccine was made part of the immunisation schedule in 1992. It is worthwhile vaccinating susceptible contacts of patients with measles as in 'vaccine-induced' measles, antibodies develop faster than they do following natural infection. Therefore it can be used to protect susceptible contacts during an outbreak. However, the antibody responses of rubella and mumps are too slow to do the same. The measles virus inhibits the body's response to tuberculin resulting in false-negative Heaf and Mantoux tests for up to one month after vaccination with MMR.

3.15   **Answers: A E**

The stepwise treatment of asthma involves starting at the 'step' most appropriate to severity and moving up or down as needed. Treatment can be gradually 'stepped down' if control has been good for over six months.

Step 1:   try occasional beta-agonists – if required more than daily then treatment should progress to include the steps below:
Step 2:   inhaled cromoglycate, nedocromil or low dose inhaled steroids
Step 3:   high dose inhaled steroids or low dose inhaled steroids plus long acting inhaled β-agonist
Step 4:   high dose inhaled steroids plus trials of inhaled long acting β-agonists, theophylline, ipratropium bromide, oral long-acting β-agonists
Step 5:   addition of regular steroid tablets

3.16   **Answers: A B E**

The gene for cystic fibrosis is located on the long arm of chromosome 7 and analysis of fetal DNA obtained in the first trimester (at chorionic villous biopsy) will confirm the diagnosis. There is a gene carrier rate of 1 in 22 of the Caucasian population and approximately 75–80% of these gene mutations in the UK are due to a deletion at delta F508, although this frequency varies geographically (e.g. in Italy, it is only responsible for about 40% of mutations).
Cystic fibrosis is an autosomal recessive disorder, therefore two carrier parents have a 1 in 2 chance of having a carrier child, a 1 in 4 chance of having a normal child and a 1 in 4 chance of having an affected child.

3.17   Answers: **A B C E**

UTIs are more common in boys in the first month of life and become more common in girls from about six months. *E. coli* is responsible for approximately 80% of cases. Other causative organisms include Klebsiella, *S. albus* and Proteus. In neonates most UTIs are haematogenous in origin, whereas in older infants and children infection generally ascends from native bowel flora. About 35% of all children presenting with a UTI have VUR, with 45% having some structural or functional abnormality of their urinary tract (90% if < two years and 60% if < five years).

Significant bacteriuria from a normal MSU or clean catch has $> 10^5$ bacteria/ml, however a suprapubic aspirate requires $> 10^3$ bacteria/ml only.

3.18   Answers: **A D E**

Infantile spasms are rare with a usual onset between four and nine months. They characteristically present with 'jack-knife' or 'salaam' attacks, which involve sudden flexion of the trunk, head and arms. These spasms typically last only a second but can recur several times a minute ('drop attacks' are characteristic of myoclonic astatic epilepsy).

The EEG shows hypsarrhythmia in 66% and 70% will have localized or diffuse brain lesions on CT scan, (tuberous sclerosis, brain malformations and chronic trauma) while 30% have no identifiable cause. The children with brain damage are refractory to treatment and develop psychomotor retardation by five years, whereas cryptogenic cases respond better to treatment – seizures settle by five years and 50% develop a normal IQ. First-line treatment is prednisolone or ACTH for three months followed by benzodiazepines or valproate.

3.19   Answers: **A C**

Generalized 'absences' present between three and 13 years and are more common in girls. 'Absences' characteristically last less than 10 seconds and recur more than 10 times a day. There is no collapse and the patient is usually unaware of them. Affected children have a normal IQ but may have learning difficulties secondary to the frequency of the attacks.

The EEG shows bilateral symmetrical 3Hz spike and wave pattern, which may be precipitated by hyperventilation (EEG spike waves over Rolandic are typical of simple partial seizures). A CT scan reveals no structural abnormality and the cause is unknown, though they may have a familial predisposition. It usually remits in adult life, but 30% go on to develop generalized tonic-clonic epilepsy. First-line treatment is with valproate or ethosuximide.

3.20   **Answers: A B C D E**

Primary generalized tonic-clonic epilepsy is rare, has no known cause and typically presents after five years of age. There is usually no aura, although these do occur in partial seizures with secondary generalization. Features include an initial tonic spasm associated with collapse, loss of consciousness and cyanosis lasting more than 60 seconds. This is usually followed by clonic spasms with incontinence and tongue biting. lasting more than three minutes. The ensuing post-ictal phase or coma gradually resolves over several minutes to hours with headache, drowsiness, confusion, myalgia and automatism.

Complications include status epilepticus which is a fit (or consecutive fits without complete recovery between) lasting more than 30 minutes. The EEG may be normal between seizures or show bursts of spike waves. During the tonic phase, diffuse runs of spike waves occur with slow waves alternating with spike waves in the clonic phase.

First-line treatment is carbamazepine, with 70% of patients being fit-free on monotherapy alone. Second-line agents include lamotrigine or valproate with phenytoin and phenobarbitone being third-line. After 15 years, 80% will remain in remission off treatment altogether.

3.21   **Answers: B D**

No vaccine is contraindicated in cerebral palsy and full immunisation should be encouraged. Feeding difficulties occur due to hypertonia and problems arise because of the persistence of primitive reflexes (e.g. Moro, grasp and the asymmetric tonic neonatal reflex).

3.22   **Answers: A C D**

Constipation is the passage of hard, dry stools resulting in distress for the child. However, it may present as diarrhoea when constipation with overflow is present. Breast-fed babies may pass infrequent soft stools (e.g. weekly), but this is a normal variation and parents should be reassured. Constipation is most commonly secondary to a low fibre diet, although other causes include: anal fissures, medication, dehydration, anal trauma (e.g. post operatively, abuse) and spinal disorders (e.g. spina bifida). Mental retardation is associated with failure to develop a regular bowel habit, however Down's syndrome is also associated with an increased incidence of Hirschsprung's disease.

3.23   **Answers: A B C**

There are certain common factors that predispose to child abuse. These include parental factors, such as coming from a broken home, possibly being abused themselves and thus lacking a suitable role model from whom to develop good parenting skills. They may have a personality disorder or be psychiatrically unwell.

Risk factors associated with the child include prematurity, especially if the child was admitted to SCBU. The ensuing maternal separation results in a three-fold risk of abuse. Other features are children resulting from an unwanted pregnancy or those with a chronic illness or behavioural problems. The great majority of children abused are under four years old. Social factors are also an issue, any family crisis (e.g. bereavement, unemployment) increases the risk of abuse. Drug/alcohol dependence, poor housing, stepchildren, maternal exhaustion and social isolation are also all features. Extended family nearby lessens the risk.

3.24   **Answers: A D E**

Pica is defined as the 'eating of things that are not food'. It is likely to be associated with other signs of disturbed behaviour or a decreased IQ. If disciplinary approaches are unsuccessful a community paediatric referral may be appropriate to assess any developmental delay. It is associated with iron deficiency anaemia although it is not fully understood how or why, but may respond to a short course of iron supplements.

The 'mouthing' of objects seen at eight months is a normal transient developmental phase. However if this persists beyond two years of age it is likely to be associated with some developmental problem.

3.25   **Answers: B C D E**

Attention deficit disorder (ADD) is the term applied to unusually overactive children with accompanying lack of concentration, impulsiveness and emotional immaturity, boys are affected more than girls in a ratio of 5:1. Various associations include lead poisoning, drugs (e.g. phenobarbitone, phenytoin and theophylline) and possibly food additives (e.g. tartrazine-E102, sunset yellow-E110, carmiosine-E122 and amaranth). Other foods that may exacerbate hyperactivity in some children include cows' milk and wheat.

ADD is diagnosed more frequently in the USA. In the UK it is felt to be uncommon in isolation, but possibly occurs more frequently in association with conduct disorders or mental retardation. Psychosocial assessment which involves counselling parents and teaching simple behaviour modification techniques is the mainstay of treatment. Medical treatment includes Ritalin and dietary advice may also have a role.

3.26   **Answers: B C D E**

Non-accidental injury should be suspected when there is a delay in presentation of the child with an inadequate or inconsistent explanation of the symptoms or lesions. An unusual parental attitude, such as over protection or alternatively appearing unconcerned should also cause concern.

Accidental skull fractures tend to be single, linear, narrow and parietal with rarely any associated intracranial injury. A depressed skull fracture is therefore highly suspicious, as is a fractured tibia in a non-ambulant child of six months. Black eyes are difficult to obtain except via a punching injury, consequently unilateral, but particularly bilateral black eyes are suggestive of abuse.

3.27   **Answers: B C D E**

The Butler-Schloss report recommends that parents should be invited to attend all or part of the conference, unless the chairman feels their presence will be detrimental to the child's interests. It should ideally be held during the EPO and a senior officer from social services must act as the chairman. Other invitees include the GP, paediatrician, police child protection team, a solicitor from the local authority and other specialists as appropriate.

The case conference acts in an advisory capacity only and considers the evidence of abuse, the cause, the risk of recurrence and safety of any siblings. However, apart from deciding whether to put the child on the Child Protection Register, all other decisions are made by the directors of social services, who will obviously take into consideration the findings of the case conference.

3.28   **Answers: A B E**

Salicylate poisoning can cause both a respiratory alkalosis and metabolic acidosis. However, while a respiratory alkalosis is a common finding in adults, children tend to have a more prominent metabolic acidosis. Hyperglycaemia is another feature of salicylate poisoning.

A serum salicylate level of < 400 mg/L is rarely symptomatic, whereas levels > 1.2 g/L are usually lethal. The mainstay of treatment involves correcting acidosis, hypoglycaemia and dehydration with i.v. fluid replacement, while ensuring a urine output of 5–6 ml/kg/hr. Urgent dialysis may be required for acute renal failure. Salicylate poisoning may also result in hypoprothrombinaemia that can cause a coagulopathy requiring correction with vitamin K and FFP.

3.29   **Answers: B E**

Features of Kawasaki syndrome include non-suppurative cervical lymphadenopathy, fever which may last several weeks with an elevated CRP, ESR and platelet count. Other characteristic signs include non-purulent conjunctivitis, changes in the oral mucous membranes, a generalised urticarial rash with swollen, erythematous hands and feet resulting in periungual desquamation after 2–3 weeks.

Coronary artery aneurysm development is a late complication and therefore an echocardiogram is not required urgently, but should be routinely performed at 2–3 weeks.

3.30   **Answers: A C D**

Reye's syndrome is acute encephalopathy with fatty degeneration of the liver, kidneys and pancreas, resulting in vomiting, delirium, fits and coma. Other features include hepatomegaly, hypoglycaemia, cerebral oedema and hyperammonaemia. The aetiology is unclear, but viral illness and aspirin exposure have been postulated as precipitating risk factors. Indeed there has been a steady decline in incidence since 1986 when aspirin was withdrawn from use in young children.

It usually presents before the age of two years after a prodromal illness and is associated with a high mortality. The transaminases are typically elevated, but the bilirubin is usually normal. Treatment involves general supportive measures and reduction of any raised intracranial pressures with normalisation of the $PaCO_2$ and i.v. mannitol. Complications include renal failure, GI bleed and pancreatitis and should be managed accordingly.

3.31   **Answers: C E**

The characteristic features of Fallot's tetralogy are a ventricular septal defect (VSD), pulmonary stenosis, an overriding aorta and ventricular hypertrophy resulting in a right to left shunt. Fallot's tetralogy together with TGA are the two leading causes of cyanotic congenital heart disease. In Fallot's tetralogy central cyanosis occurs with infundibular spasm which is relieved by propranolol.

There is no murmur associated with the VSD, however the pulmonary stenosis typically results in an ejection systolic murmur heard best over the pulmonary area. The characteristic CXR appearance of Fallot's tetralogy is a 'boot shaped' cardiac shadow, whereas the 'egg on its side' is more typical of TGA.

3.32 **Answers: A B**

Coarctation of the aorta involves narrowing of the aorta. It is five times more common in males and is also associated with Turner's syndrome. Aortic constriction leads to radio femoral pulse delay, a higher BP in the arms than in the legs and an ejection systolic murmur heard over the precordium and between the scapulae. The CXR may reveal a visible indentation at the site of the coarctation and cardiomegaly in severe cases. The classic 'rib-notching' resulting from accessory vessel formation develops in older children.

Early presentation is associated with a more severe narrowing and higher mortality, whereas older children may present as an incidental finding on routine examination. Surgical correction aims to lessen the risk of developing endocarditis and hypertension and should always be performed.

3.33 **Answers: A D**

Congenital heart disease (CHD) has an incidence of 8 per 1000 live births with VSD being the most common. Acyanotic lesions (e.g. VSD, ASD, PDA and pulmonary stenosis) are approximately three times more common than cyanotic lesions (e.g. TGA and Fallot's) and generally have a better prognosis.

Down's syndrome is associated with an increased incidence of VSD and ASD. Other risk factors for CHD include maternal drug and alcohol abuse, maternal diabetes, maternal infection (e.g. rubella), a positive family history and Turner's syndrome (e.g. coarctation).

Indomethacin is a prostaglandin synthetase inhibitor and may lead to premature closure of the ductus. In TGA, i.v. prostaglandin E is given to keep the ductus open until urgent catheterization can be carried out. Definitive surgery is postponed until about nine to 12 months.

3.34 **Answers: B C**

Torsion of the testis presents between 14 to 20 years of age with symptoms of acute scrotal, lower abdominal or even hip pain. Predisposing factors include maldescent, a long mesorchium and high riding, horizontally positioned testes. They are not associated with inguinal herniae. Torsion of the testes is a surgical emergency, 80% are viable if operated on within five hours, but after 24 hours 100% of testes have infarcted. USS is a useful investigation, but should not delay surgical exploration, which is the only definitive method of confirming the diagnosis. The opposite testis should be fixed at the same time.

3.35   **Answer: A**

Vasoconstriction of the ophthalmic artery occurs in simple migraine resulting in transient visual aura, scintillating scotoma, zigzag lines (fortification phenomena), visual field defects and micropsia. Strabismus, diplopia and nystagmus are all signs of possible intracranial pathology. Papilloedema is a sign of raised intracranial pressure indicating more serious intracranial pathology.

3.36   **Answers: A C E**

Edward's syndrome (trisomy 18) is associated with hypertonicity, low set malformed ears, receding chin, protruding eyes, cleft lip/palate, rocker bottom feet and umbilical/inguinal herniae. Expected survival is approximately ten months.

Laurence–Moon–Biedl is an autosomal recessive condition that mainly affects boys. It presents with night blindness, progressing to visual loss. Other features include obesity, polydactyly, small genitals, paraparesis, decreased IQ, retinitis pigmentosa, squint and cataract.

Noonan's syndrome is an autosomal dominant condition with a 1 in 5000 prevalence. Any system may be affected, but common associations include heart defects (e.g. hypertrophic cardiomyopathy/septal defects), ptosis, downward slanting eyes, low set ears and a webbed neck. There may be a coagulopathy and slightly reduced height and IQ.

Pierre Robin syndrome is neonatal difficulty with feeding and breathing secondary to micrognathia (short chin) ± cleft palate.

Turner's syndrome (XO) has a prevalence of 1 in 2500 girls and is associated with short stature, a wide carrying angle (cubitus valgus), webbed neck, coarctation of the aorta and rudimentary or absent gonads.

3.37 **Answers: A E**

Features of nephrotic syndrome include proteinuria, hypoalbuminaemia, generalised oedema and hyperlipidaemia. The serum albumin should be < 25 g/l with proteinuria > 1 g/m^2/24 hours. Peak incidence is between two and five years of age with the majority being due to 'minimal change glomerulonephritis'. This accounts for 70–80% of cases of primary nephrotic syndrome. It has an incidence of approximately 2 in 100,000 in the UK with a male: female ratio of 2:1. Over 90% respond to steroid therapy.

Diffuse proliferative glomerulonephritis accounts for approximately 10% of cases of primary nephrotic syndrome (focal segmental – 10%; membranous – 2%). Other causes of nephrotic syndrome include congenital and secondary causes (e.g. collagen disorders, diabetes mellitus, toxins).

Initial management involves hospital admission for assessment and treatment. This may include corticosteroids, antibiotics, fluid management and diuretics. A high protein, no salt diet is poorly tolerated and adequate proteins will be provided with a normal balanced diet. Salt restriction is only used if there is progressive oedema.

3.38 **Answers: C D E**

Tuberculin testing traditionally involves an injection into the flexor surface of the left forearm. The Heaf test is ideally read at seven days (between 3–10 days) and the Mantoux test is read at 48–72 hours (but up to 96 hours). A positive result occurs when the area of induration is > 5 mm. N.B. the area of 'flare' is irrelevant. The Heaf test is graded 0–4. Heaf grade 0–1 is negative and grade 2–4 is positive. Strongly positive reactions (i.e. Heaf grade 3–4 or induration > 15 mm) require further investigation and possible antituberculous chemotherapy.

3.39 **Answers: A B C**

Down's syndrome is the leading cause of severe learning difficulties. It affects approximately 1 in 660 births. Trisomy 21 is responsible for 90% of cases and has a recurrence risk of about 1%. The incidence increases with maternal age, with woman of 40 years having a 1 in 40 risk.

Typical features include developmental delay with an IQ between 20 and 75. They have a characteristic appearance of up-slanting eyes with wide epicanthic folds, a small nose with a low bridge, a small mouth with a protruding tongue, a single palmar crease and general hypotonia/ joint laxity. 40% have a cardiac lesion particularly a PDA or ASD. Other common disorders include duodenal atresia, thyroid disease and leukaemia.

3.40   **Answers: A B C E**

Rickets is the inadequate mineralization of new bone in developing bones (osteomalacia in adults). It is most commonly secondary to vitamin D deficiency (e.g. diet, malabsorption or lack of exposure to sunlight). Other associations include chronic renal failure and anti-convulsant therapy, as phenytoin and phenobarbitone induce liver enzymes resulting in accelerated breakdown of cholecalciferol to its inactive metabolite. Inherited causes include vitamin D dependent (autosomal recessive) and vitamin D resistant (X-linked dominant trait) rickets.

Clinical features include frontal bossing, kyphoscoliosis, hypotonia, swelling at the wrist and costochondral junctions ('rickety rosary'). Bow legs (genu varum) are more usual in toddlers, whereas knock-knees (genu valgum) are typical of older children. Tetany and convulsions secondary to hypocalcaemia may occur rarely.

Treatment of nutritional rickets involves parental education and high dose vitamin D supplements for 4–6 weeks, then low dose until biochemical and radiological resolution.

3.41   **Answers: C D**

Predisposing features for iron deficiency anaemia include low birth weight, prematurity, the early introduction of cows' milk, blood loss (e.g. Meckel's, parasites i.e. hookworm), and malabsorption (e.g. coeliac, *Giardia*).

A blood film shows a hypochromic, microcytic picture with target cells. Serum iron and ferritin are low and the TIBC is raised. Treatment involves correcting the underlying cause, dietary advice and iron supplementation for approximately eight weeks. A reticulocyte peak between 5–10 days and an increase in haemoglobin (by 2 g/dl every three weeks) can assess an adequate response to treatment.

3.42 **Answers: A B**

Haemoglobin is made of two α and two β chains. In thalassaemia there is a defect in the genes responsible for their manufacture. In thalassaemia major both β chain genes are affected, whereas only one is affected in thalassaemia minor. β-thalassaemia is most commonly found amongst the Mediterranean races, but also in Burma and Thailand.

Thalassaemia minor rarely causes problems, however thalassaemia major presents with failure to thrive, clinical anaemia and poor feeding from about six months of age. Other features include hepatosplenomegaly and bone changes, secondary to the associated marrow hyperplasia, such as frontal bossing and generalized osteoporosis.

Typically there is a hypochromic microcytic blood film with target cells, the TIBC is normal and serum ferritin is markedly elevated. Management involves regular blood transfusions with the iron-chelating agent, desferrioxamine, in order to prevent haemosiderosis from the associated excessive iron storage. A splenectomy may be required if there is evidence of hypersplenism (i.e. excessive transfusion requirements, gross splenomegaly and/or thrombocytopenia). This results in an increased risk of pneumococcal infection and therefore requires vaccination ± prophylactic penicillin. Folic acid supplements are also recommended.

3.43 **Answers: A C D E**

Sickle cell anaemia is an autosomal recessive condition that results from synthesis of an abnormal Hb chain (HBs). It is common amongst the Negro races with HBs carriage occurring in 40% of black Africans and 10% of UK Afro-Caribbeans. It can be diagnosed via fetal blood sampling at around 18/40 or earlier from fetal DNA analysis of cells from amniotic fluid or trophoblast biopsy.

Heterozygotes (sickle cell trait) are usually asymptomatic unless severely hypoxic and typically have a normal haemoglobin and blood film. Homozygotes (sickle cell disease) however, present with acute haemolysis and frequent painful sickling crises of mainly fingers and toes from about six months, and larger joints from three to four years. Their haemoglobin is usually around 6–8 g/dl and their blood films typically show hypochromia, target cells, Howell–Jolly bodies and occasional sickle cells. The associated chronic haemolytic anaemia results in an increased incidence of pigment gallstones leading to biliary colic.

Management involves treating the underlying cause and supportive measures using fluids, oxygen and analgesia. Antibiotics, blood or even exchange transfusion may also be necessary acutely. Splenectomy should be considered for hypersplenism or recurrent sequestration crises and should always be covered with pneumococcal vaccination ± prophylactic penicillin.

3.44   Answers: B C D E

Both haemophilia A and B are X-linked disorders and result from deficient factor VIII coagulation. In both conditions the intrinsic clotting pathway is affected resulting in a prolonged APTR. The prothrombin time measures the extrinsic pathway and is therefore normal. Haemophilia presents with an increased risk of haemorrhage, resulting in bruising, recurrent haemarthroses (leading to progressive joint destruction) and following surgery or dental extraction rendering prophylactic dental care essential.

Management of acute bleeds requires the prompt administration of factor VIII concentrate (or cryoprecipitate/fresh frozen plasma). Patients must never receive aspirin or be given intramuscular injections and a haematological opinion should be sought prior to any surgical procedure.

3.45   Answers: B C E

G6PD deficiency is an X-linked condition and globally is the commonest enzyme deficiency known. There are three main genetic variants – Mediterranean, African and Oriental. Diminished activity of the enzyme G6PD results in a red cell that is more susceptible to oxidants leading to acute episodes of haemolysis. This has many precipitants, such as infection/illness; drugs (e.g. antimalarials, antibiotics – sulphonamides, nitrofurantoin); and fava beans (Mediterranean and Oriental types only). During a crises the haemoglobin may be 2–5 g/dl and the blood film shows crescent cells, spherocytes and Heinz bodies (Howell–Jolly bodies occur post-splenectomy). Between crises there is no anaemia, the blood film is normal and diagnosis must be made on enzyme assays.

Management involves avoiding precipitants, good hydration, blood transfusion for severe anaemia, analgesia and occasionally the use of antioxidants, such as methylene blue or vitamin C.

3.46   Answers: A C D E

3.47   Answers: A B D E

Acute lymphoblastic leukaemia has a 50–75% five-year disease-free survival rate, but approximately 10% relapse within the first year. Poor prognostic features include age < 2 years or > 10 years, a presenting WCC > 20,000 mm^3, T or B cell surface markers, elevated acid phosphatase in T-cell leukaemia, an anterior mediastinal mass or CNS signs at presentation. Being Caucasian is a good prognostic factor.

3.48 **Answers: A B**

In the UK, cows' milk protein intolerance is the most common cause of chronic diarrhoea in infants under one year of age. Other common causes include constipation with overflow, post gastroenteritis (e.g. lactose intolerance), infections (e.g. salmonella, giardia) and toddler diarrhoea which is suggested by recognizable food in the stool, is of unknown cause and is not of any sinister significance.

Coeliac disease is due to sensitivity to gluten in wheat and rye, which causes the characteristic jejunal villous atrophy seen at biopsy and leads to malabsorption. However, this is not diagnostic, as similar appearances may be found with gastroenteritis and cows' milk intolerance. Diagnosis is confirmed by clinical remission within weeks of commencing a gluten-free diet and associated reduction in the number of circulating IgA specific antibodies. It has an incidence of about 1 in 2000 and tends to run in families with girls being more commonly affected. It usually presents at between nine months and three years with failure to thrive and frequent loose stool, although mild cases may remain undiagnosed into adulthood.

Diffuse inflammation and ulceration of the colon characterise ulcerative colitis; it is rare in childhood and is not inherited in a Mendelian fashion.

3.49 **Answers: C E**

Indications for tonsillectomy include recurrent febrile convulsions associated with attacks of follicular tonsillitis; over three attacks of bacterial tonsillitis in two consecutive years and tonsils that are so grossly enlarged in between infections that they meet in the midline causing stridor or sleep apnoea. Primary post-op haemorrhage occurs within 24 hours and is usually due to inadequate haemostasis, whereas secondary haemorrhage occurs between 7–10 days and is commonly due to infection. Purulent follicular exudate may occur in both bacterial and viral tonsillitis. Some authorities claim that bacterial infection requires at least ten days antimicrobial treatment, although there is little evidence for this in industrialised societies.

Adenoidectomy is a useful treatment for glue ear, as the adenoids may encroach upon the nasopharyngeal orifice of the Eustachian tube. It can be performed at the same time as grommet insertion and myringotomy.

3.50   **Answers: A E**

Acute otitis media is caused by a viral infection in over 50% of cases, the remainder are usually due to *Haemophilus influenzae*, Group A haemolytic, streptococci and pneumococci. Amoxycillin is the treatment of choice, with cephalexin and erythromycin being second line. Referral to an ENT surgeon should be considered for children having three or more episodes in a year.

There may well be bullous formation on the eardrum, however this is not associated with any particular organism and needs no treatment apart from that of the acute infection. One month following an attack 40% of affected children have no effusion and at three months 90% are clear.

3.51   **Answers: A B D E**

Appendicitis is rare in the under fives, but nearly 90% of cases present with perforation demonstrating the difficulty in diagnosis. Problems may be due to the child's ineloquent history and because of its rarity it is not thought of initially. Also, small abdomens may make localising pain in the RIF difficult to elicit. Retrocaecal appendicitis may not cause any localising signs (PR reveals tenderness anteriorly) or the child may present with urinary symptoms/signs if a pelvic appendix is inflamed. A useful sign is the child's ability to 'hop' or 'jump' as peritonitis is excluded if this is painless, making the diagnoses of appendicitis unlikely. Differential diagnoses include mesenteric adenitis, UTI, DKA, intussusception, lower lobe pneumonia and infectious hepatitis.

3.52   **Answers: A B**

The Health Visitor relieves the midwife of responsibility at ten days post delivery and is subsequently responsible for child health surveillance in all children up to five years of age. They are informed of every child under five that attends A&E and are then obliged to contact the parents/guardians for appropriate follow-up. They also supervise the running of immunization clinics, however social workers are responsible for children in care.

3.53   **Answers: B C D E**

Language delay has an increased occurrence amongst boys and children from large families – with first born and only children being the least likely to be affected. Other associated features include developmental delay, deafness, autism and abnormalities of the speech apparatus i.e. neurological (e.g. cerebral palsy) and physical (e.g. cleft palate – this is secondary to dysarthria and recurrent otitis media). Severe language delay has as an incidence of 1 in 1000.

Speech therapists can accurately assess children between one and five years using the Reynals developmental language scale, to see whether the delay is due to comprehension, expression or both. Management depends on the cause and may involve a multidisciplinary approach, including audiology, orthodontic referral, plastic surgery or simply speech therapy alone.

3.54   **Answers: A D**

Crohn's disease is characterised by inflammation of the whole thickness of the bowel, especially the terminal ileum and proximal colon, the rectum is usually spared. The incidence has increased over the last 20–30 years and now affects about 5 per 100,000 individuals. Presenting features include failure to thrive, mouth ulcers, anorexia, abdominal pain and diarrhoea. Other non-GI features include erythema nodosum, arthritis, digital clubbing and anaemia. Investigations include a malabsorption and infection screen, endoscopy, biopsy and barium meal, which may reveal the characteristic 'string sign', 'skip lesion' and 'rose thorn ulcers' seen in Crohn's disease.

Ulcerative colitis classically has diffuse inflammation and ulceration of the entire rectal and colonic mucosa and is also associated with an incidence of 5 per 100,000. It typically presents within the first 12 months or around ten years of age with intermittent episodes of abdominal pain and bloody diarrhoea. Other features include lethargy, fever, clubbing, mouth ulcers, anaemia, arthritis, short stature, erythema nodosum and toxic dilatation of the colon. Investigations include malabsorption and infection screens, double contrast barium enema, colonoscopy and biopsies.

Management for both involves a high-energy, low-fibre diet with vitamin supplements and drugs (e.g. mesalazine or sulphathalazine) associated with immunosuppressive agents, such as steroids. Surgery is indicated in Crohn's only if there are complications such as bowel obstruction or perforation. However, in ulcerative colitis, surgery may be required for failure to respond to conservative treatment, toxic dilatation, severe GI bleed, perforation and ultimately as prophylaxis against its associated increased risk of malignancy.

3.55   **Answers: B D**

Precocious puberty is defined as the onset of sexual maturation before eight years in a girl and nine years in a boy. It is at least four times more common in girls and usually no cause is found. However, in boys it is essential to investigate as in 80–90% of cases a cause is found (e.g. intracranial tumour). The most important sequelae is a decreased final height, as the initial associated growth spurt is short lived, because the advanced bone age results in early epiphyseal fusion.

Important investigations include a skull X-ray, bone age, CT scan of the head, urinary 17-ketosteroids, pelvic USS and thyroid function tests. Management involves referral to a specialist for treatment aiming to achieve continually high levels of synthetic GnRH analogues in the circulation. This 'non-pulsatile' regime paradoxically suppresses the secretion of pituitary gonadotrophins, which reverses gonadal and slows skeletal maturation. Treatment should be continued until the average age of puberty (i.e. 11 years) and parents should be reassured that the child will develop normally.

Features of McCune–Albright syndrome include polyosteotic fibrous dysplasia of bone, irregular areas of skin pigmentation, facial asymmetry ± precocious puberty. Coeliac disease is associated with delayed puberty.

3.56   **Answers: A B E**

Anorexia nervosa occurs predominantly amongst teenage girls, affecting 1 in 250 between the ages of 15 to 18 years, although boys represent up to 5% of cases. Features include persistent refusal to eat leading to potentially dangerous weight loss, intense fear of becoming obese, disturbed perception of body image and primary or secondary amenorrhoea due to endocrine disturbance (low LH, FSH and oestrogen). N.B. Amenorrhoea before weight loss should arouse suspicion of hypothalamic dysfunction.

Symptoms may include excessive exercise, laxative/diuretic abuse and induction of vomiting which may result in hypokalaemia. Other physical complications include sensitivity to cold, constipation, faints, lethargy, hypotension and hypoglycaemia.

The aetiology is multifactorial with family dynamics a key issue. Management involves gaining the patient's trust, outpatient psychotherapy for mild cases and admission in severe cases for treatment of medical complications, family therapy, individual psychotherapy including privileges for weight gain and occasionally drugs (e.g. anxiolytics, antidepressants). Depression and suicide attempts are common. Approximately 50% remain underweight with psychological difficulties and the overall mortality rates are up to 8%.

3.57   **Answers: D E**

Low birth weight (LBW) babies are those weighing < 2500 g, whereas very low birth weight (VLBW) babies weigh < 1500 g. Together they account for approximately 1 in 15 infants born in the UK. A LBW infant may be small for gestational age (SGA) i.e. < 10th centile, premature i.e. born before 37/40 or both.

SGA babies may reflect maternal factors, such as chronic illness (e.g. CRF), hypertension, smoking, alcohol and undernutrition which results in placental insufficiency and thus intrauterine growth retardation (IUGR). Maternal diabetes typically results in 'large for dates' babies. Problems include an increased incidence of congenital malformations, intrapartum asphyxia, hypoglycaemia, impaired thermoregulation, respiratory distress syndrome in premature infants and jaundice. Survival has improved over the years with over 95% of infants born weighing 2000–2500 g surviving and only about 8% of surviving infants suffering a major handicap (e.g. cerebral palsy).

3.58   **Answer: B**

Bow legs are normal in infants and usually correct by three years of age. Knock knees (genu valgum) are normal up to approximately five years. Predisposing conditions include osteogenesis imperfecta, rickets, Blount's disease (infantile tibia vara) and chondrodysplasia. Genu varum also results from medial tibial torsion, this usually spontaneously corrects within five years and no treatment is required. However, forward bowing is pathological (e.g. rickets) and active management is essential.

Osgood–Schlatter's disease occurs with inflammation of the tibial tuberosity at the insertion of the patella tendon and results in painful knees. Neither bow legs nor knock knees are a feature, although the latter is a common sequela of poliomyelitis.

3.59   **Answers: C D E**

Neisseria gonorrhoeae may cause ophthalmia neonatorum, however *Chlamydia* is more frequently responsible. Stevens–Johnson syndrome is a systemic disorder associated with erythema multiforme ('target' lesions), fever, mouth, genital and eye ulcers.

Orbital cellulitis presents with significant orbital oedema, limitation of ocular movements, fever and altered colour vision as a late feature. Causes include adjacent sinusitis, bacteraemia and other local infection. Intrauterine infections which predispose to neonatal cataracts include toxoplasmosis, rubella, cytomegalovirus (CMV), herpes simplex and varicella. Other causes include autosomal inheritance and chromosomal disorders (e.g. Down's syndrome), metabolic disorders (e.g. diabetes mellitus), trauma and the use of systemic steroids.

Glaucoma is rare in childhood and results from defective drainage of aqueous humour from the anterior chamber. It may be due to primary causes such as aniridia or secondary causes such as iritis, trauma or intraocular tumour.

3.60   **Answers: B C D E**

An MCU should not be performed acutely, as transient reflux may occur following a bladder infection and the MCU also risks introducing infection. Thus, it should ideally be deferred for a few weeks following a UTI and then always under antibiotic cover. DMSA is taken up by functioning renal tubular epithelial cells and shows areas of renal parenchymal damage i.e. 'scars'. DTPA is processed by the kidney in the same way as inulin and is therefore good at assessing the differential function of the kidneys.

All children less than one year should be investigated with an AXR, USS, DMSA and MCU after their first infection. Children between one and six years require an USS and DMSA. A MCU is only performed if the previous investigations are abnormal; if the first infection was pyelonephritis; if the UTIs are recurrent or there is a family history of chronic atrophic pyelonephritis. Children over six years require investigation with an USS only after their first UTI.

1. *List the pros and cons in performing a splenectomy on a child with a hereditary spherocytosis. Outline your long-term management.*

Advantages

Prevention of:
- Anaemia and jaundice by reducing the excessive haemolysis – although spherocytosis will still persist
- Gallstones from raised bile salts secondary to elevated haemoglobin metabolism
- Leg ulcers
- Aplastic crises which are generally precipitated by a viral infection particularly parvovirus
- Megaloblastic crisis resulting from folate depletion due to hyperactivity of the bone marrow
- Removal of splenomegaly

The spleen should be removed in all but the mildest cases, although it may be deferred in children due to the risk of infection. The decision to perform a splenectomy is hard if asymptomatic, but a raised bilirubin and especially the presence of gallstones are strong indications. Alternative treatment may include folic acid supplements and transfusions for haemolytic and aplastic crises.

Disadvantages

- The risks associated with having a general anaesthetic and major surgery.
- Immediately post-operatively there is an elevated platelet count (generally 600–1000 x 10^9/L) which lasts for 2–3 weeks putting the patient at a risk of thromboembolic phenomena.
- There is an increased risk of overwhelming infection especially pneumococcal and parasitic infections (especially falciparum malaria).

Long term treatment

- All children should be given prophylactic penicillin (250 mg/bd)
- All should receive polyvalent anti-pneumococcal vaccine (preferably given 2-3 weeks pre-operatively). Hib vaccine is also recommended and possibly meningococcal vaccine.
- Malarial prophylaxis is necessary when travelling to high risk countries
- Full blood count and folate levels should be checked regularly and long-term follow-up is vital.

2. ***Discuss 'cyanotic breath holding' attacks. What advice would you give mother?***

Breath holding attacks occur between the ages of six months and five years. The child when thwarted or hurt cries, then holds its breath in expiration, turns blue and after 10–15 seconds goes limp. He may lose consciousness and generally when this happens a normal breathing pattern is resumed and a pink colour returns.

If breath holding continues for a further 10–15 seconds a convulsion may ensue, this may be differentiated from an epileptic convulsion in which the cry is synchronous with tonic phase and cyanosis occurs late, and which is neally always 'spontaneous'.

Management

- Involves taking a careful history and examination to establish the diagnosis – the latter is expected to be normal.
- It is important to discuss the mother's anxieties about the diagnosis and potential management plans.
- You may be able to instruct the mother in methods of distraction which when used may terminate an episode early.
- It is vital to set the limits of allowable behaviour and to stress the importance of a firm and consistent handling if these limits are exceeded.
- Finally reassure the mother that the child will outgrow the habit by about 4-5 years of age.

3. **What features would make you suspect a non-accidental injury in a toddler with a periorbital bruise? What are the aims of a Child Protection Case Conference?**

A periorbital haematoma is a suspected wound

- It is important to determine if there has been any delay in presentation
- Have the parents provided a reasonable explanation of the injury and is this consistent on further questioning?
- Does the child have other injuries or failure to thrive?
  Is he unkempt, frightened or withdrawn?
  Does he have 'frozen watchfulness'?
  Is there a history of developmental retardation?
- Observe the parental attitude to the child e.g. is there abnormal interaction, aggression, reluctance to allow a full examination or derogatory comments?
- Have there been multiple consultations in the past about minor symptoms?
- Do the parents express fear of damaging the child or an inability to cope?
- Is the toddler (or any of his siblings) on the child protection register?

Parental factors may also be important

- Do they lack personal experience of good parenting skills and family support?
- The risk to the child is increased 20-fold if the parents themselves were abused.
- Do the parents suffer from personality disorders or psychiatric illness and do they have unreasonable expectations of the child?

Factors pertaining to the child

- Was the child the result of an unwanted pregnancy?
- Were there neonatal problems e.g. a premature baby has a threefold risk of being abused
- Does the child have a birth defect or is it the 'wrong sex'
- Is it a difficult child suffering from chronic illness, feeding or sleep problems?

Social factors

- Family crises e.g. marital, unemployment, eviction, bereavement, drug and alcohol dependence, poor housing, debt, isolation, frequent pregnancies, maternal exhaustion or depression
- Change in family structure e.g. step children are at increased risk
- Do they come from a violent society, where aggressive behaviour is almost the norm?.

The aims of a case conference are to:

- Share all relevant information and review evidence of abuse, possible aetiology and the likelihood of recurrence
- Assess the safety of the child/children in a family and to decide whether legal action is required to protect them
- Obtain legal advice as to whether legal action is likely to succeed
- Decide whether their names should be added to the 'child protection register'
- Devise a plan for future work, including assessment of the needs of the family and what help is available locally
- Nominate a key worker
- Recommend follow-up and case review

Apart from the decision about registration the case conference acts in an advisory capacity only. Decisions are the responsibility of the Directors of Social Services who will take recommendations of the case conference into account.

The parents should also be invited to attend all or part of the conference unless the Chairman feels that their presence will preclude proper consideration of the child's interests.

4.   *Write short notes on unilateral cryptorchidism.*

Testicles should have descended by 36 weeks gestation and therefore cryptorchidism is associated with prematurity. Occurring in 100% of boys born at less than 32 weeks, approximately 3% at term and 0.5% at 1 year of age. In 25% of cases both testes are undescended although generally the right is more commonly undescended as the left testis begins its descent into the scrotum first.

The aetiology is unknown and the testes generally lie along the path of normal descent, often near the external inguinal ring. The testis is generally smaller than average and often impalpable and if not in the scrotum by four years of age will result in spermatic tubule and germ cell atrophy. The child's ipsilateral scrotum is frequently poorly developed and may be associated with renal abnormalities (may need IVP/renal USS etc).

Complications

- Include malignant tumours; the incidence is 0.3/1000 of scrotal testes, 10/1000 of groin testes and 50/1000 of abdominal testes.
- The diagnosis of testicular neoplasia is also made much later as the testes are not palpable and thus so is the tumour, resulting in a worse prognisis.
- Up to 30% of boys with unilateral cryptorchidism may become sub-fertile (60% of bilateral cases are infertile) due to impaired spermatogenesis.
- Following orchidopexy some testes atrophy and HRT may be needed in adolescence.
- The incidence of torsion is increased.

Management

- The mal-descent should be noted and follow-up arranged at three months (correcting for gestation)
- If still undescended at this time the child will need referral for orchidopexy (after one year spontaneous descent will not occur). Orchidopexy is then performed around the age of two years and no later than four years.
- HCG may cause descent, in 30% of bilateral and 15% of unilateral cases but surgery is more successful at preserving fertility.

5. **What is cerebral palsy? Outline different methods of its classification.**

Cerebral palsy is a disorder of posture and movement resulting from a non-progressive lesion of the developing brain before or during the neonatal period. The expression of the lesion changes as the brain matures.

Classification as 'movement disorder'

- Spasticity (i.e. lesion in cortex or internal capsule) is an increase in muscle tone
- Dyskinetic (i.e. lesion in the basal ganglia) is a collective term for several different movement disorders such as:
  chorea (abrupt, jerky movements)
  athetosis (slow, writhing, continual movement of the extremities)
  dystonia (writhing movement leading to sustained bizarre posturing of the trunk and extremities)
- Ataxic (i.e. lesion in the cerebellum) is an incoordination of movement
- There may also be a mixed picture

Classification by 'cause'

The cause of cerebral palsy is unknown in about 40-60% of cases. However, in approximately 20-30% of patients there is correlation with various risk factors, such as:

Prenatal
- Cerebral malformation
- Intra-uterine infection
- Metabolic defect
- Obstetric complications
- Chronic anaemia

Perinatal
- Hypoxic ischaemic injury
- Complications of extreme prematurity e.g. PVH
- Metabolic causes i.e. kernicterus/hypoglycaemia, neonatal meningitis

Post-natal
- CNS infection
- Trauma
- Hypoxia
- Diplegia: the lower limbs are more affected than the upper limbs
- Hemiplegia: one side of the body is more affected than the other (and the arm is usually more affected than the ipsilateral leg)
- Quadriplegia: all four limbs are similarly affected
- Paraplegia: both legs are affected but the arms are spared

NB. Associated problems of cerebral palsy include: strabismus; language and learning difficulties, hearing loss, developmental delay and behavioural problems; epilepsy.

6. ***An 11-month-old girl presents with a 7 hour history of screaming episodes approximately every 20 minutes appearing calm between attacks. Discuss your management of the most likely diagnosis.***

Probable diagnosis

- Intussusception requiring emergency admission.

Management

- Firstly ensure that the airway, breathing and circulation are stable.

History

- Take a full history including ante-natal, birth, SCBU and any other hospital admissions.
- Ask about associated symptoms i.e. diarrhoea and vomiting, appetite, weight loss or gain, fevers and rashes. Is the child passing urine? If there is diarrhoea is it watery or loose, has the child opened his bowels or is he constipated? Has he passed mucus, pus, fresh blood or redcurrant jelly per rectum.
- Is there any family history of similar episodes?

Examination

- Do a full examination including temperature, lymphadenopathy, dehydration (fontanelle, mucous membranes, skin)
- Check the cardiovascular system for evidence of shock or collapse (e.g. tachycardia, slow capillary return, hypotension)
- Do a neurological examination looking at tone, symmetry, meningism
- Gastro-intestinal system examination:
  Is the abdomen soft, tender, is there guarding and rebound?
  Is there any organomegaly?
  Are there any masses on palpation (sausage shaped)?
  Are bowel sounds present?
  Do a rectal examination and look at the child's nappies for further clues (i.e. presence of blood/mucous)

Investigation

- Urinalysis
- Full blood count
- Urea, electrolytes and creatinine
- Supine abdominal X-ray +/- chest X-ray (? free gas under diaphragm)
- Abdominal ultrasound scan
- Enema (air/barium) which may be diagnostic and therapeutic

Treatment

- Intravenous fluid replacement
- Diagnostic/therapeutic enema
- Abdominal surgery for peritonitis or failed hydrostatic reduction

7.   What is the differential diagnosis of a 10-month-old child presenting with fresh blood on the surface of his stools. How would you manage this case?

Differential diagnosis

- Constipation/anal fissures
- Meckel's diverticulum (generally causes melaena)
- 'Gut' infection e.g. Campylobacter, Shigella, Salmonella, Giardia
- Inflammatory bowel disorders i.e. Crohn's, ulcerative colitis
- Foreign body/trauma
- Physical/sexual abuse
- Haematological disorders i.e. ITP/coagulopathies

MANAGEMENT

History

- Is the child well or unwell, when did it start, has he had it before, does he have constipation or diarrhoea?
- Is there any anorexia, lethargy, general pain, vomiting, fevers, pain on opening his bowels or weight loss?
- Is there a history of foreign travel or recent change in diet etc?
- Take a past medical history including development and any previous hospital admissions
- Take a family history including inflammatory bowel disease, bleeding tendencies and a history of atopy or cows' milk intolerance

Examination

- Perform a full examination assessing the general appearance of the child, monitor the centile charts and look for signs of disease including fever, dehydration, anaemia, jaundice, mouth ulcers, clubbing (generally occurs after 12 months), bruising and lymphadenopathy
- Abdominal examination should look for tenderness, guarding, bowel sounds, organomegaly and other masses, the presence of inflammation around the anus with or without fissures, or fistulae, finally perform a rectal examination looking for further masses and examine the stool (soft/hard; blood/mucus?)

Investigations

- Urinalysis for blood
- Microscopy, culture and sensitivities of stool (and urine if dipstix positive)
- Faecal occult blood
- Malabsorption screen (full blood count/film, ESR, U&Es, LFTs serum ferritin) total IgE and specific IgE to milk/eggs etc.
- Abdominal X-ray
- Barium meal/enema
- Endo/colonoscopy +/- biopsy

Treatment

- Of the infection includes oral rehydration therapy or if associated with abdominal pain or severe vomiting then intravenous fluid replacement may be more appropriate +/- antibiotics as indicated
- Of inflammatory bowel disease includes steroids (oral/enemas) diet, surgery and psychological support
- Of anal fissures depends on the cause, this is normally secondary to constipation, therefore diet modification +/- osmotic/stimulant laxatives, +/- enemas/glycerine suppositories, +/- manual evacuation under GA

8. Write short notes on school refusal versus truancy.

	SCHOOL REFUSAL	**TRUANCY**
Age	5–11 years	8 years and over
Previous school attendance	Normally good – used to enjoy	Poor – dislikes school
Family	Generally a conventional cohesive family which may collude over the non-attendance. It is usually a small family from social class 1-3	Generally a large family who are unaware or are unconcerned and tend to come from social class 4-5
Personality	The child is normally conscientious, conforming and anxious	The child is normally rebellious and anti-social
Achievement	Good with high goals	Non-academic with only practical goals
Psychosomatic features	Common	Rare
Triggers	Accidents, illness and bereavement	Domestic crisis, change of school
Sex	Girls = Boys	Boys > Girls
IQ	High	Low
Prognosis	Better	Poorer
Parents	Tend to be over-protective and anxious	Disinterested, inconsistent discipline with corporal punishment
Father	Not strongly supportive	There is a history of absence
History of separations e.g. recurrent hospital admissions	Fewer	More

9.   *A toddler develops a febrile illness. On examination a murmur is heard on auscultation. What features imply it is not significant?*

- A systolic (mid) murmur (any diastolic component is unlikely to be innocent)
- Soft/buzzing in character and short in duration
- Absence of a thrill
- Heard at the left sternal edge without radiation
- The child is otherwise well with normal growth and is otherwise active i.e. no evidence of aortic stenosis, clubbing, heart failure etc.
- The heart sounds normal with no other associated features such as clicks, thrills, diastolic components or radiation
- The murmur has never been heard before, i.e. it is not previously recorded in the medical notes
- The pulses are normal, no femoral delay
- The murmur is variable i.e. if it increases in intensity on exercise or fluctuates with different positions
- The murmur is specifically associated with the febrile illness and resolves with recovery from infection

10a.   *What factors predispose to iron deficiency in the under two-year-olds?*

Dietary factors are the most common cause of anaemia with the maximum incidence occurring between six months and three years of age. Infants have an increased susceptibility because more than 75% of the total iron in neonates is in the circulating haemoglobin. Therefore stores are dependent on the haemoglobin concentration at birth and the blood volume. In addition, breast milk has a low iron content.

Stores of iron in term infants are sufficient for approximately four months normal requirements. From 4-12 months a daily oral intake of greater than 1 mg/kg of elemental iron is needed (assuming absorption efficiency is approximately 10%).

Premature and low birth weight infants will have inadequate stores at birth and will therefore need supplements until established on a mixed diet.

The predisposing dietary factors to anaemia include
- Low birth weight/prematurity
- Inappropriate early introduction of unmodified (cows') milk
- Prolonged breast feeding
- Delayed weaning
- No supplements
- Poor diet

Other non-dietary factors include
- Malabsorption e.g. coeliac disease
- Blood loss
- Chronic illness

10b.   Is screening for iron deficiency beneficial and how would you go about it?

Screening for iron deficiency is beneficial in preventing poor growth and developmental delay. It is a relatively easy and cheap test to do and requires minimal training. It is a common condition in the UK which can be treated simply with dietary advice and supplements.

Screening can be performed while the child is having other routine checks or immunisations e.g. with the MMR at 12-18 months. Establishing a history of poor diet and lethargy and noting the child is pale with koilonychia etc. on examination can be followed up with a simple finger prick blood test.

However, there is no national policy in the UK.

CASE COMMENTARY 1

1. Discuss the possible differential diagnoses and assess her failure to thrive?

A differential diagnosis includes:

- A slow growing but otherwise normal, healthy infant
- An underfed healthy infant
- An emotionally deprived but reasonably well fed infant
- A chronically ill infant e.g. cystic fibrosis
- A physically or mentally abnormal infant
- An infant with malabsorption e.g. coeliac disease or cows' milk protein intolerance

Jane's assessment includes a full history, examination and investigations. The history should include any antenatal problems. The fact that she was premature and ventilated leads to a three-fold increase in the risk of child abuse, probably due to impairment in bonding. Did she reach her other milestones on time and is there any past medical history of note resulting in multiple hospital admissions and parental separations? Was this a planned pregnancy and did they want twins? Does she have any behavioural problems e.g. difficulty feeding/sleeping, or chronic illness? Jane's dietary history is also important.

Other risk factors include the fact that the parents are both young, have a low income, are facing unemployment with increased financial stress and possible eviction. They have three children under three years of age, which is a high risk factor for maternal exhaustion and depression and as a full time housewife she gets no respite from her children. Ask about any marital difficulties or any drug/alcohol abuse. Do they have any support nearby from friends or family or has their recent move left them in social isolation?

A full examination is necessary, looking for signs of abuse and parental attitude towards Jane. Check her head circumference, height, weight on her centile charts and assess whether she has lost weight recently or has always been underweight. If the parent-held child health record is available, then growth velocity can be assessed with more useful data. A neurological examination is also important to assess for any residual deficit secondary to her cerebral insult and a complete developmental examination is particularly important in assessing if there is global delay or just motor delay. Initial investigations should be simple and may include urinalysis and culture, stool culture, FBC, CRP, U&Es, creatinine, serum ferritin +/- coeliac antibody screen.

2. **Differentiate the various possible reasons for her inability to walk.**
93–95% of delayed walking is idiopathic; as Jane has significant medical problems then delayed gross motor development should be expected. Unrecognised problems identified because of her late walking include:

- Mild cerebral palsy (neurological examination may show hypotonia, brisk reflexes, difficulty with dorsiflexion of her feet and a mild hemi, as well as diplegia)
- Mild global learning difficulties (fine motor/language developmental delay)
- Psycho-social deprivation (ascertained from the history)
- She may have a primary muscle disorder and if a male child consider Duchenne muscular dystrophy (CPK blood levels, muscle biopsy)
- Missed congenital hip dislocation

3. **Outline methods of helping this family**
Copies of Jane's previous medical and neonatal records should be obtained and a period as an inpatient should be considered to observe feeding, stools, parental skills etc. A multi-disciplinary review should be organised and appropriate follow-up arranged. They should be encouraged to draw upon their extended family for support and inform them of other areas of support available e.g. individual psychotherapy, family therapy to aid bonding, family centres and telephone help lines etc. Financial advice may also be appropriate and the availability of child care facilities.

CASE COMMENTARY 2

1. Describe her cough and how you would investigate it.
The cough is not typical of any known disease process including asthma although this cannot be totally disregarded; it is likely to be 'hysterical'. Investigations should include a full history as to the nature of the cough, is it productive or non-productive? Is there any other precipitating factors other than stress? Does it actually stop her from doing anything? Is it associated with breathing difficulties? Does she feel otherwise 'well'? etc.

A drug history should also be taken for any medication (prescribed or otherwise) that might precipitate a cough or other substances that cause coughs e.g. cigarettes. Is there a family history of atopy or any past medical history of note?

The social history should include an assessment of the family dynamics. Are there any marital or financial stresses? Has there been a recent bereavement or illness? A school report would also be helpful (with the parents' permission). Does she have friends? Has her schoolwork been deteriorating?

A full examination is also vital including a thorough respiratory examination. Some simple investigations are appropriate and should include a peak expiratory flow rate, oxygen saturation and sputum culture and if in any clinical doubt a chest X-ray. In the first instance limit the investigations as overdoing it can lead to anxiety in Chloe and her parents that there is actually something physically wrong.

2. How would you investigate her poor appetite?
Chloe is extremely underweight with no evidence of illness or malabsorption and she has almost certainly developed severe anorexia nervosa. However, organic disease should also be excluded. Initial investigations as always should include a history. Is it just food, or does drinking also result in abdominal distension? Are any particular foods associated and is there any diarrhoea or vomiting? Does she admit to any of the physical symptoms related to severe mal-nourishment e.g. tiredness, fainting, dizziness, feeling cold and constipation etc.? Does she calorie count? Does she have any phobias? What is her body image and what does she want to be when she grows up? e.g. ballet dancer/model. Is there a family history of obesity, anorexia or bowel disorders?

A full examination is necessary including a thorough abdominal examination looking for signs of malnutrition and anorexia (thin, lethargic, hypothermia, bradycardia, peripheral cyanosis, and lanugo hair). Is she wearing baggy clothes to conceal her weight loss? Review her centile charts for height and weight.

Initial investigation should include full blood count, urea and electrolytes, glucose, a stool sample for culture and faecal fat and a urine specimen for culture and the presence of ketones. Depending on the diagnosis being investigated other tests may be more suitable e.g. coeliac serological screen.

3. What would you discuss with Chloe and her parents at this point?
Chloe has many risk factors for having anorexia nervosa. She is a ballet dancer, has a high IQ, comes from social class 1–2 and has an anxious personality. Ask about any family stresses or school stresses that may have triggered this condition. Are any friends at school 'dieting'? Does Chloe have a pre-morbid personality? i.e. emotionally immature, obsessive traits, ambivalent mother/child relationship. It is important to emphasise the health risks that she is exposing herself to, and point out how she may have fewer physical symptoms at a higher body weight. Explain that the probable diagnosis is anorexia nervosa and ask them how they feel about that.

4. What strategies would you use to assist Chloe?
Establish a rapport with Chloe and her family and refer early to the local child guidance specialist with an interest in anorexia for outpatients' 'psychological management'. In Chloe's case inpatient management may be more appropriate initially with sessions in individual and family therapy and strict regimens of e.g. privileges for weight gain. Resistant anorexia nervosa or deterioration also needs urgent admission to hospital.

There is a high rate of child sexual abuse in this group and this must be considered. It is important to interview Chloe on her own once her confidence has been gained to explore this issue. Regular follow up is also vital, setting goals of gradual weight gain under the direction of a specialist dietician. Drug therapy may also be useful i.e. anxiolytics and antidepressants.

THE CLINICAL EXAMINATION

INTRODUCTION

It is important to read the College guidelines for the clinical part of the DCH examination. These can be obtained from the Royal College of Paediatrics and Child Health direct or downloaded from the College web site. The guidelines set out the syllabus for the exam, the format, what is expected in the clinical section in general and specific guidelines relating to developmental assessment and child health surveillance.

It is of particular importance to read the following sections:

- Vision, visual disorders and visual testing in the DCH examination
- Guidelines for hearing testing in the DCH clinicals
- Language development guidelines
- Child Health Surveillance: knowledge and standards for the DCH examination
- Psychiatric guidelines

The format of the clinical exam is one Long Case, where 40 minutes are spent with the patient and 20 minutes with the examiners, followed by several Short Cases over 30 minutes, of which 10 minutes are devoted to developmental testing, including the testing of vision and hearing.

The guidelines state that standard equipment appropriate to the examination will be provided. A stethoscope should be taken. You may prefer to take other objects with which you are familiar, such as an ophthalmoscope and developmental kit.

Remember that the clinical examination tests your ability to

- take a good case history
- perform a competent physical examination
- recognise abnormal physical signs
- assess growth and development
- assess the special senses
- assess psychiatric status

THE LONG CASE

It is essential to get a clear medical history but also to concentrate on the social, behavioural, family and educational issues of the case. Use a checklist to make sure you don't miss out anything out:

- Presenting complaint
- History of presenting complaint
- Past medical history including birth history
- Immunisations
- Developmental history including behaviour and educational issues
- Drugs history and allergies
- Social history
- Family history
- Review of systems to check you haven't missed anything out

Perform a complete physical examination including assessment of growth and development.

- Practise seeing the child in the appropriate time
- Practise presenting and think out and practice answers to questions on the long case
- Practise problem orientated presentation

This means presenting the patient clearly, listing active and inactive problems with the aim of giving the examiner an overview of the case in the first few sentences.

Allocate your time carefully allowing time to collect your thoughts, think about the case and prepare the case for presentation to the examiners.

Examples of Problem Orientated Presentation

Case One

A 6-year-old girl presents with Down's syndrome. She has recently been diagnosed as hypothyroid. She is on treatment and well at the moment. Her other problems are

- Obesity
- Constipation
- Previous surgery for Hirschsprung's disease
- Learning difficulties
- Social and family issues

It may be that the entire discussion focuses on the learning difficulties and how her schooling is sorted out.

This includes

- Pre-school learning support including portage
- Statement of special education needs
- Review of special educational needs

and requires knowledge of the assessment of children with special educational needs which can be found in any of the standard community paediatric texts.

Alternatively the examiner could focus on the medical complications seen in a child with Down's syndrome:

- Cardiac problems
- Hypothyroidism, other auto-immune problems
- Hirschsprung's disease
- Atlanto-axial instability
- Leukaemia

Alternatively the examiner could spend most of the time discussing specific emotional issues:

- How have the child's problems affected the parents and the other siblings? What has been the effect on the integrity of the family unit?

Children with cerebral palsy are often seen and the case can be presented in a systematic and organised way in the same manner.

Case Two

An 8-year-old boy presents with cerebral palsy. He has a spastic quadriplegia and is in a wheelchair. His main problems are

- Difficulties with feeding, poor weight gain and recurrent chest infections
- Fits which are well controlled on anticonvulsant therapy
- Joint contractures and poor mobility
- Difficulties with schooling
- Social and family issues

It may be that you then go on to discuss either the medical aspects of this child's care or the multidisciplinary management. It is important to remember this list.

Professionals potentially involved in the multidisciplinary management of an 8-year-old with a spastic quadriplegia:

- Occupational therapist
- Speech and language therapist
- Dietician
- Teacher
- Educational psychologist
- Social worker
- General Practitioner
- Community paediatrician
- Orthopaedic surgeon

This list could be applied to many other long cases.

Case Three

An 8-month-old child presents with bronchopulmonary dysplasia. His condition is stable at the moment. His main problems are

- Chronic chest disease requiring home oxygen
- Severe failure to thrive – nasogastric tube feed dependant
- Pre-term – 25 weeks gestation – with delayed motor development
- Social problems

The subsequent discussion may focus on one or all of these problems. Nutritional assessment will be of obvious concern and the reasons for his failure to thrive and the potential action that can be taken to overcome it may be discussed. Alternatively the social situation could be focused on, with discussion about why there may be problems.

Examples of Long Cases

Any condition may be seen and it is important not to be too put off if you don't know too much about the case that you see. Concentrate on putting the case together well and giving a well thought out multidisciplinary presentation.

Asthma
Cerebral palsy
Ex-premature baby with chronic lung disease
Cystic fibrosis
Spina bifida
Down's syndrome
Neurofibromatosis
Crohn's disease
Coeliac disease
Nephrotic syndrome
Chronic renal failure
Cyanotic congenital heart disease
Marfan's syndrome
Undiagnosed short stature
Prader-Willi syndrome
Muscular dystrophy

SHORT CASES

It is essential to have a clear scheme for the examination of potential scenarios you might meet in the exam and a good knowledge base of the common conditions which you might see. This section outlines some of this with lists of commonly seen cases and should be used as a revision checklist in the preparation for the clinical part of the exam.

The section does not duplicate the information listed in the DCH handbook relating to the examination of special senses (see above)

- Practise how you would deal with the listed common short cases
- Practise interacting with the child and parent. Introduce yourself.
- Practise presentation skills. Make some initial comments. State what you can see, for example if you think someone might have Down's syndrome say so. Otherwise the examiner won't know. The same goes for things like a nasogastric tube, drip etc. If you see something obvious say so.
- Practise talking through the examination
- Team up with a like-minded candidate and practise presenting cases to each other

Basic format for clinical examination

- Be prepared to talk about your findings as you go on
- Introduce yourself to the child and parent
- Look
- Feel
- Listen
- Describe your findings
- Answer questions about them as you walk over to the next short case

EXAMINATION OF CARDIOVASCULAR SYSTEM

Look
- Dysmorphic features e.g. Down's syndrome (VSD), Turner's syndrome (coarctation), Noonan's syndrome (pulmonary stenosis)
- Is the child thriving?
- Respiratory distress, cyanosis

Hands
- Pulse – brachial is better in babies, check for radio-femoral delay
- Clubbing
- Peripheral cyanosis

Blood pressure
- Mention but don't necessarily do (but be prepared to if asked)

Face
- Anaemia
- Central cyanosis

Neck
- JVP (older child)

Scars
- Cardiac catheterisation scars
- Thoracotomy scars, e.g. shunt procedure, PDA ligation, coarctation repair
- Central sternotomy scars, e.g. corrective procedures (VSD repair, ASD repair, Tetralogy of Fallot repair, arterial switch for repair of transposition of the great arteries) or palliative procedures, e.g. shunt

Palpation
- Apex beat – including localisation, presence of heaves – check for dextrocardia
- Thrills – include supra-sternal thrill and carotid thrill

Auscultation
Listen in the four areas
- Mitral (apex)
- Tricuspid (left sternal edge)
- Aortic (right second intercostal space)
- Pulmonary (left second intercostal space)
- And for radiation

Heart sounds
- Are they present?
- Is the second heart sound normal – loud (pulmonary hypertension), split (ASD), single (aortic stenosis)?
- Click (aortic stenosis, pulmonary stenosis)

Murmurs
- Timing in relation to cardiac cycle
- Systolic/diastolic/continuous/mixed systolic and diastolic 'to and fro'
- Grade
- Site of maximal intensity, radiation (neck, axilla and back)
- Character
- Murmur enhancing moves – left lateral position, sitting forward

Grading of Murmurs
I   barely audible
I   medium intensity
III loud but no thrill
IV   loud with a thrill
V   very loud but still requires stethoscope to be on the chest
VI   so loud, heard with stethoscope off the chest

Further examination
- Do not forget anything you may have left until the end e.g. blood pressure, femoral pulses
- Listen to the back for murmurs
- Palpate the liver

Common Short Cases – Cardiology

Innocent murmur
Ventricular septal defect
Atrioventricular septal defect
Atrial septal defect
Pulmonary stenosis
Aortic stenosis
Coarctation of the aorta
Dextrocardia – may be associated situs inversus
Cyanosed child who may or may not have had cardiac surgery
Eisenmenger's syndrome

Remember, children whose heart disease has been repaired may be seen and that chest wall scars may not be present, for example a child who has had a balloon dilatation of pulmonary stenosis by cardiac catheter.

EXAMINATION OF RESPIRATORY SYSTEM

Look
- Is the child thriving, inhalers/nebulisers, pancreatic enzymes, peak flow meter, sputum pot?
- Is the child obviously hyperexpanded?
- Is the child in respiratory distress?

Hands
- Clubbing, cyanosis and anaemia
- Count pulse and respiratory rate

Respiratory effort
- Examine for pectus excavatum and Harrison's sulci
- Nasal flaring, recession, tracheal tug

Mouth
- Central cyanosis

Chest
- Scars
- Feel suprasternal notch for tracheal deviation, palpate apex beat (mediastinal shift)
- Percuss (anteriorly, posteriorly and lateral)
- Listen (anteriorly, posteriorly and lateral)

At the end of your examination
- Ask to examine the ears, nose and throat, see sputum specimen and perform peak flow measurement (if appropriate)
- Assess for tactile vocal fremitus, vocal resonance if appropriate (e.g. suspected consolidation)

In a baby it may be reasonable to change the order of examination to gain the maximum information.

Remember the common causes of clubbing

Congenital
Cyanotic congenital heart disease
Bacterial endocarditis
Cystic fibrosis
Bronchiectasis
Chronic active hepatitis
Inflammatory bowel disease

Hyperexpansion

This implies chest disease and is an extremely important physical sign. Practise the assessment of hyperexpansion. Look from the front first and then assess by looking at the child from the side and examining antero-posterior diameter and its excursion during the respiratory phases. Comment on asymmetry if seen.

Causes of hyperexpansion – common conditions seen in the exam

- Asthma
- Bronchopulmonary dysplasia- look for neonatal sequelae e.g. head shape, chest drain/iv scars
- Cystic fibrosis
- Bronchiectasis

Harrison's sulcus

Harrison's sulcus is visible as a bilateral fixed indrawing of the anterior portion of the lower ribs. It is caused by chronic airway obstruction encouraging excessive diaphragmatic use which causes deformity where the diaphragm inserts into the rib-cage. Its presence therefore suggests long-standing airway obstruction.

Hyperexpanded chest plus clubbing implies cystic fibrosis or bronchiectasis

Hyperexpanded chest without clubbing implies asthma or bronchopulmonary dysplasia

Pectus Carinatum = prominent sternum
Pectus Excavatum = sternal depression

GASTRO-INTESTINAL EXAMINATION

Remember gastro-intestinal examination will pick up gastro-intestinal, renal and haematological pathology.

Look
- Does the child look well?
- Normal or dysmorphic
- Nasogastric tube, iv cannula
- Well nourished (adequate exposure) – comment on nutritional status
- Mention the need to plot on a growth chart

Hands
- Clubbing
- Koilonychia
- Palmar erythema
- Pallor

Eyes
- Jaundice
- Anaemia

Mouth
- Peri-oral pigmentation – Peutz-Jeghers syndrome
- Mouth ulceration
- Tongue – stomatitis
- Teeth

Chest
- Spider naevi
- Gynaecomastia

Abdomen
- Scars (laparoscope, groin, loin)
- Umbilical hernia
- Abnormal vessels – caput medusae (drain from the umbilicus)
- Distension
- Superficial palpation – all over once
- Deep palpation – all over once
- Liver
- Spleen
- Kidneys

Further examination

This should be done as appropriate and depends on the previous findings. For example it is not necessary to look for shifting dullness if the abdomen is not distended.

- Percussion
- Bowel sounds
- Abdominal distension – stand child up and look at buttocks as may also be wasted suggesting malabsorption
- Ascites – fluid thrill, shifting dullness – only if distended
- Can I see the back?
- Can I see the genitalia?
- Hernia orifices

Common Short Cases – Gastro-intestinal examination

Abdominal scars
Gastrostomy tube
Cystic fibrosis
Crohn's disease
Coeliac disease
Constipation
Umbilical hernia
Hepatomegaly, splenomegaly and hepatosplenomegaly
Glycogen and other storage disorders
Portal hypertension,
Hereditary spherocytosis
Sickle cell disease,
Thalassaemia
Mucopolysaccharidoses
Post Kasai for biliary atresia
Liver transplant
Nephrotic syndrome
Steroid toxicity
Renal masses

Examination of the liver, spleen and kidneys

- Important to do correctly
- Liver/spleen – start in right iliac fossa
- If organomegaly found, confirm with percussion – measure if appropriate

Liver
- Edge – regular or irregular?
- Surface – smooth or nodular?
- Texture – firm or hard?
- Tenderness
- Is there a rub?
- Is there a bruit?

Spleen
- As above
- ?Hepatomegaly and ascites
- Associations e.g. jaundice – hereditary spherocytosis

Common exam questions

How do you differentiate between a liver, spleen and kidney?
Why is it a liver ?
Why is it a spleen ?

Liver
- Right hypochondrium
- Cannot get above it
- Moves with respiration
- Dull to percussion

Spleen
- Left hypochondrium
- Cannot get above it
- Moves with respiration
- Dull to percussion
- Has a notch

Kidney
- Can get above it
- Doesn't move with respiration
- Resonant
- Ballotable

EXAMINATION OF THE THYROID GLAND

Need a glass of water (may be beside the bed). Start by making general comments – does the child look well, do they seem appropriately grown?

Look
- Look from the front with the neck extended for enlargement of the thyroid gland
- Is the enlargement uniform or unilateral?
- Ask the child to take a drink – thyroid swelling should move upwards with swallowing
- Ask child to stick tongue out. A thyroglossal cyst will move upwards.

Palpate
- Palpate the gland whilst standing behind the child
- Assess size, shape consistency and surface of the mass
- Again ask to drink whilst palpating

Also
- Palpate for lymphadenopathy
- Percuss sternum for retro-sternal extension
- Auscultate for bruits

Scheme For examination of thyroid status

- Look generally at the child. Comment on growth.
- Feel hands – warm and sweaty (hyperthyroid) or cold and blue (hypothyroid)
- Ask to hold arms outstretched for fine tremor (hyperthyroid)
- Count pulse – tachycardia (hyperthyroid), bradycardia (hypothyroid)
- Take blood pressure (wide pulse pressure in hyperthyroidism)
- Examine eyes for exophthalmos and lid lag (Grave's disease)
- Examine cardiovascular system for flow murmurs and hyperactive praecordium (hyperthyroidism)
- Examine abdomen for constipation (hypothyroid)
- Examine for a proximal myopathy (hyper or hypothyroidism)
- Pre-tibial oedema (hypothyroidism)
- Tendon reflexes (hypothyroidism – slow relaxation)

EXAMINATION OF A SHORT CHILD

Offer to plot height. Ask about previous heights. Ask about parental heights. Note pubertal status – may be obvious e.g. post pubertal female.

1.   Is the child obviously dysmorphic?

e.g. Turner's syndrome, Noonan's syndrome, Russell-Silver dwarfism, Prader-Willi syndrome. If so then direct the examination towards that problem.

2.   Does the child have a skeletal dysplasia?

e.g. achondroplasia, hypochondroplasia, spondyloepiphyseal dysplasia.

3.   Is there an obvious systemic disease?

Thin child – e.g. cystic fibrosis/bronchiectasis, coeliac disease, inflammatory bowel disease

Fat child – e.g. cushingoid, hypothyroidism, hypopituitarism/growth hormone deficiency

4.   Consider other possibilities

- Constitutional delay
- Familial short stature
- Emotional/food deprivation

INTERPRETING PARENTAL HEIGHT

Expected centile = (mother's height centile + father's height centile)/2

Expected final adult height

BOY   (father's height + (mother's height +12.5 cm))/2

GIRL   ((father's height - 12.5 cm)+mother's height)/2

Tall Stature

Tall children and adolescents are frequently seen; remember the potential causes including familial tall stature, tall stature secondary to obesity and Marfan's syndrome.

EXAMINATION OF THE SKIN

This is difficult and it is not possible to have a scheme which is always applicable.

- Aim for good exposure
- Look at the hands, nails and wrists
- Look at the elbows
- Exposure of other areas (front and back)
- Look at the child from head to toe including mouth and teeth
- If desperate ask if there is a rash and where it is
- Recognise common disorders

Common Short Cases – Dermatology

Eczema
Strawberry naevus
Mongolian blue spot
Psoriasis
Capillary haemangioma
Café au lait spots (neurofibromatosis)
Sebaceous naevus
Vitiligo
Lipodystrophies
Molluscum contagiosum
Epidermolysis bullosa
Ectodermal dysplasia
Henoch-Schönlein purpura

EXAMINATION OF THE JOINTS

Look
- General appearance of the child
- Any obvious clues e.g. orthoses, shoes, splints
- Look for any deformity, erythema, swelling around the joint, scars from previous infection or surgery
- Look at muscle bulk
- Compare with normal joint

Feel
- Watch patient's face while palpating the joint
- Feel for skin temperature, tenderness, and joint effusion

Move
Ask the child to move the joint before you move it to ensure that movement is not painful and to get some idea of the range of movement possible. It is important to do this as you don't want to cause pain as soon as you touch the patient!

Function
Assess the function of the joint if possible e.g. ask the child to walk, pick up an object etc

- Use one of the larger texts to read about the examination of individual joints

Common Short Cases – Rheumatology

Perthes' disease
Juvenile chronic arthritis
Psoriatic arthritis
Juvenile dermatomyositis
Haemophilia
Osteogenesis imperfecta
Congenital dislocation of the hip
Toe walking
Hemihypertrophy

DEVELOPMENTAL ASSESSMENT

Remember the areas of development
- Gross Motor
- Fine Motor and Vision
- Speech and Hearing
- Social

In the assessment of a child's development in the exam it is essential to discuss milestones from each of these four areas.

MILESTONES

It is essential to learn a list of developmental milestones. A selection of milestones is listed below.

6 WEEKS

Gross motor	holds chin up when prone, beginning to lose head lag
Fine motor and vision	follows object up to 180 degrees in the horizontal plane, watches people
Social	smiles

12 WEEKS

Gross motor	lifts head and chest with extended arms when prone, reaches forward, but misses objects, supine early head control, loss of Moro reflex, makes defensive movements
Fine motor and vision	fixes and follows in the horizontal and vertical plane
Social	sustained social contact, listens to music, begins to vocalise

16 WEEKS

Gross motor	lifts head and chest into vertical axis, legs extended, hands in midline, reaches and grasps objects and brings them to the mouth. No head lag on pulling to the sitting position. Held erect, pushes with feet.
Social	laughs out loud, shows displeasure, excited at sight of food

28 WEEKS

Gross motor
rolls over prone to supine (first) then supine to prone, sits with rounded back and leans forward on hands, supports most of weight on standing and bounces actively, reaches out and grasps for large objects, transfers from hand to hand, grasps using radial grasp, rakes at pellets

Speech and hearing
polysyllabic vowel sounds formed

Social
prefers mother, babbles, enjoys mirror

40 WEEKS

Gross motor
sits alone without support, back straight, pulls to standing position and cruises around the furniture, creeps and crawls

Fine motor and vision
grasps objects with thumb and forefinger, pokes at things with a forefinger, picks up a pellet with assisted pincer grip (using radial border of arm), uncovers hidden toy, object permanence

Speech and hearing
repetitive consonant sounds mama, dada, should pass distraction test (see later)

Social
responds to sound of name, plays peek-a-boo or pat-a-cake, waves bye-bye

1 YEAR

Gross motor
walks with one hand held, rises independently

Fine motor and vision
full pincer grip, releases objects on request

Speech and hearing
few words besides mama, dada, beginning to have meaning

Social
plays simple ball game, makes postural adjustments to dressing

15 MONTHS

Gross motor
walks alone, crawls upstairs

Fine motor and vision
makes tower 3 cubes, makes line with crayon, inserts pellet into bottle

Speech and hearing
jargon, may name familiar objects

Social
hugs parents, indicates desires and needs

18 MONTHS

Gross motor	runs stiffly, sits on small chair, walks upstairs with hand held, explores
Fine motor and vision	tower of 4 cubes, imitates scribbling, imitates vertical strokes, dumps pellet
Speech and hearing	10 words, names pictures, identifies one or more body parts
Social	feeds self, seeks help, tells when wet/soiled, kisses parents with pucker

2 YEARS

Gross motor	runs well, walks up and down stairs one step at a time, opens doors, climbs on furniture, jumps
Fine motor and vision	tower 7 cubes, circular scribbling, imitates horizontal strokes
Speech and hearing	puts 3 words together (subject, verb, object)
Social	handles spoon well, listens to stories, tells immediate experiences, helps to undress

2½ YEARS

Gross motor	upstairs alternating feet
Fine motor and vision	tower 9 cubes, vertical and horizontal strokes but not yet a cross, forms closed figure
Speech and hearing	refers to self as I, uses proper name
Social	helps put things away, pretends in play

3 YEARS

Gross motor	rides tricycle, stands on one foot momentarily
Fine motor and vision	tower 10 cubes, imitates bridge of 3 cubes, copies circle, imitates cross
Speech and hearing	knows age and sex, counts 3 objects correctly, repeats 3 numbers
Social	plays simple games in parallel with other children, helps in dressing, washes hands

4 YEARS

Gross motor	hops on one foot, throws ball over hand, uses scissors to cut out picture, climbs well
Fine motor and vision	copies bridge from model, imitates construction of gate from 5 cubes, copies cross and square, draws a man with 2 to 4 parts without the head
Speech and hearing	counts 4 pennies accurately, tells a story
Social	plays with other children with beginning of social interaction, goes to toilet alone

5 YEARS

Gross motor	skips
Fine motor and vision	draws triangle from copy, names heavier of 2 weights
Speech and hearing	names 4 colours, repeats sentence of 10 syllables, counts 10 pennies correctly
Social	dresses and undresses, asks questions about the meaning of words, domestic role-playing

Common Short Cases – Child Development

It is essential to practice the assessment of development and the assessment of the special senses.

Think about the following scenarios and devise a plan for the assessment incorporating the four areas of development (see above):

Six-month old – Assess this child's development
Twelve-month old – Assess this child's development
2½ years – Assess this child's development
Pre-school child – Assess this child's development
Assess this 2-year-old with delayed walking
Assess this 3-year-old who is not yet talking
Assess this 18-month-old whose parents are worried because he can't hear

Remember to use the College guidelines for assessment of hearing, assessment of vision and child health surveillance.

Use one of the community paediatric text-books for more information.

SCHEME FOR EXAMINATION OF THE CRANIAL NERVES

- Enquire about sense of smell, be prepared to examine formally if requested
- Test visual acuity
- Comment on any obvious abnormality such as squint and go on to examine formally if present
- Examine visual fields
- Examine eye movements
- Check for nystagmus – present at extremes of gaze
- Test the sensory divisions of the trigeminal nerve
- Test the motor component of the trigeminal nerve
- Test the facial nerve
- Test the auricular nerve grossly by asking the child if they can hear a very quiet noise that you make in each ear. Offer and know how to test formally.
- The glossopharyngeal nerve can be tested by the gag reflex. This should not be attempted in the exam but do mention it. Remember that the gag reflex tests the glossopharyngeal (sensory) and vagal (motor) nerves. Ask the child to say 'ah' and look at the soft palate. A lesion of the vagus causes the palate on the contralateral side to be drawn upwards.
- Test the hypoglossal nerve by asking the patient to stick out their tongue and move it from side to side
- Test accessory nerve by forced rotation of the head against resistance to check for Sternomastoid weakness

At the end of the examination you should ask to

- Look at fundi
- Assess pupillary responses to light and accommodation, offer to check corneal (V) and gag (IX) reflexes

SCHEME FOR EXAMINATION OF THE EYES

- Look at the child for any obvious clues e.g. squint, ptosis
- Does the child wear glasses?
- Look at the eyes – conjunctiva, pupils, lids
- Can the child see? – test both eyes – visual acuity
- Visual fields
- Eye movements
- Check for nystagmus
- Accommodation
- Pupil responses – direct and consensual light reflexes
- Cover test for squint
- Fundoscopy

Squint is a commonly asked topic and it is important to go to an orthoptic clinic and revise the examination of squint and be confident about it.

Convex glasses correct long sighted-ness.
Long sight = difficulty with near vision

Concave glasses correct short sighted-ness.
Short sight = difficulty with distant vision

SCHEME FOR EXAMINATION OF THE PERIPHERAL MOTOR SYSTEM

Infants

Most information is gained by observation and so spend some time watching and playing with the infant. Try to get eye contact – see if the child will fix and follow in the horizontal and vertical planes. Look for any obvious dysmorphology. Assess spontaneous movement.

- Pull the child to sit – use one hand to pull up both hands and the other to support the head
- Hold the child by the trunk in the sitting position and assess standing posture
- Hold the child up prone looking at tone and head control
- Place the child on the bed prone to see if the child supports its head, supports itself on its forearms (3 months) or outstretched hands (6 months)
- Proceed with further examination dependent upon the initial findings

Remember that if the head is extended when the child is held prone this may reflect extensor spasm and that head control is better assessed by pulling the child to sit.

Proceed to examine the tendon reflexes as you would in an older child.

Consider checking for primitive reflexes. e.g. Moro, asymmetric tonic neck reflex, grasp etc. if appropriate.

Older children

Ask the child to walk first, unless there is an obvious reason why they can't (e.g. in a wheel-chair).

- Look at muscle bulk, symmetry and for scars e.g. tendo-Achilles shortening
- Examine tone – include testing for clonus
- Examine power
- Examine reflexes
- Further examination as appropriate

Upper motor neurone or lower motor neurone lesions

Characteristics of an upper motor neurone lesion
- Increased tone
- Clonus
- Reduced power
- Increased reflexes

Characteristics of a lower motor neurone lesion
- Wasting
- Reduced tone
- Fasciculation
- Reduced power
- Reduced reflexes

EXAMINATION OF GAIT

Abnormalities to be looked for are

- Hemiplegia
- Diplegia
- Ataxia
- Lower motor neurone problem
- Myopathy
- Orthopaedic problems/rheumatological disorders

General points

First check with the child or parents that they can walk. Look at the child, do they look dysmorphic, is there an obvious cerebral palsy, is there a built up shoe, are there sticks or a wheel chair nearby?

Spastic gait

Ask the child to walk unaided – look at arm and leg movement for signs of a hemiplegia. The arm will be flexed on the affected side. If you suspect hemiplegia ask the child to walk fast or walk on tip-toe which will make the neurology more pronounced. Continue looking – are the legs stiff and abducted? If so a diplegia is likely, a diplegia will also become more pronounced if you ask the child to walk fast or on tip-toe.

Ataxic gait

If the gait is not spastic the next thing to consider is whether it is ataxic (unsteady and broad based). Ask the child to heel to toe walk (you will need to demonstrate this). If the child is ataxic this will be difficult. Then ask the child to stand and to close their eyes. If the lesion is cerebellar there should be no deterioration. If the ataxia is as a consequence of a dorsal column problem the child will fall (Romberg's sign).

Neuromuscular problem

The next possibility is that you are dealing with either a neuromuscular or a lower motor neurone problem. Look for a waddling gait and foot drop. Examine for Gower's sign.

Others

Consider either an orthopaedic or a rheumatological problem.

SCHEME FOR CEREBELLAR EXAMINATION

- Test eye movements and look for nystagmus – horizontal and maximal looking to the side of the lesion
- Ask the child a question and listen for dysarthria
- Test co-ordination. Ask the child to touch his finger then your nose with his index finger. Look for past pointing or intention tremor. Assess rapidly alternating movements (dysdiadochokinesia).
- Examine the arms and legs for hypotonia and hyporeflexia
- Ask the child to sit to check for truncal ataxia
- Stand the child up and examine for Romberg's sign to differentiate dorsal column from cerebellar disease
- Think of the causes of ataxia and look for associated signs e.g. telangiectasia (Ataxia telangiectasia) or pes cavus (Friedreich's Ataxia)

Common Short Cases – Neurology

Cerebral palsy
- Hemiplegia
- Diplegia
- Quadriplegia
- Ataxic
- Athetoid

Neuromuscular disease (older child)
- Duchenne muscular dystrophy
- Kugelberg Welander disease
- Dermatomyositis
- Peroneal muscular atrophy

The floppy infant
- Werdnig-Hoffman disease
- Myotonic dystrophy
- Down's syndrome
- Failure to thrive

Spina bifida

Ataxia
- Friedreich's ataxia
- Ataxia telangiectasia
- Ataxic cerebral palsy

Neurocutaneous syndromes
- Neurofibromatosis
- Tuberous sclerosis
- Sturge Weber syndrome

MCQ INDEX

Numbers given refer to the relevant question number. The word shown may not always be used in the question, but may appear in the explanatory answer.

MCQ Index

BIBLIOGRAPHY

ABC of One to Seven, Valman B, BMJ Books, 4th edition 1997.

ABC of Otolaryngology, Ludman H, BMJ Books, 4th edition 1997.

ABC The Firs Year of Life, Valman B, BMJ Books 4th edition 1995.

Advanced Paediatric Life Support:, Advanced Life Support Group, British Medical Association 1997.

ATLS Course Manual, Levy B.

Concise System of Orthopaedics and Fractures, Apley G, Soloman L, Butterworth Heinemann, 2nd edition 1994.

Immunisations Against Infectious Diseases, Department of Health, HMSO, 1996.

Manual of Community Paediatrics, Polnay L, Churchill Livingstone 1996.

NMS Paediatrics, Dworkin P H, Lippincott, Williams, Wilkins 2000.

Notes for the DCH, Gilbertson N J, Walker S J, Churchill Livingstone 1993.

Oxford Handbook of A&E Medicine, Wyatt J P, Illingworth R N, Oxford University Press 1999.

Oxford Handbook of Clinical Medicine, Hope A, Longmore J M, Oxford University Press 1999.

Oxford Handbook of Clinical Specialities, Collier J A B, Longmore J M, Oxford University Press, 1999.

Royal College of Surgeons STEP Course for MRCS

Paediatrics (A Primary Care Approach (STARS)), Berkowitz C D, Harcourt Health Science, 1996.

Short Cases for the Paediatric Membership, Beattie M, Clark A, Smith A, PasTest, 1999.